The Cure For Cancer

THE CURE

FOR

CANCER

BY

TERRY COOKSEY

COVER ART

BY

TERRY COOKSEY

ISBN-13: 978-1-939147-21-9
ISBN-10:   1-939147-21-2

The Cure For Cancer

THE CURE FOR CANCER

BY
TERRY COOKSEY

Table of Contents

ISBN-13: 978-1-939147-21-9

ISBN-10:   1-939147-21-2

All Rights Reserved – 2012 © American Publishing US

The Cure For Cancer

1 - Laying the Foundation for Your Cure

Yes, there is a cure for cancer. But like all cures, the cure for cancer is outside the helpless medical profession. The cure for cancer is not a gimmick. The cure for cancer is proven science that all doctors COULD tell you but don't. Your doctor only cares about prolonging your illness to maximize his income. But almost all of you will say that your doctor is different, and that he or she really cares! OK, I'll play along. But let's get some proof that your doctor really cares.

If your doctor cares, he would have told you what caused your cancer. Here's how that caring doctor conversation went. Your doctor told you that your cancer was caused by poisons, and told you this:

Cancer is caused by damage to the nucleus of cells. This damage interferes with apoptosis, which is the natural programmed death of cells. When this process breaks down, cancer cells begin to form. Cancer cells do not experience programmed death as normal cells do. This allows cancer cells to grow and divide; which leads to a mass of abnormal cells that grows out of control and forms tumors.

Once these tumors form, they develop blood vessels. These blood vessels carry cancer cells to other parts of the body and form growths. The damage to cells is caused by gene mutations causing cells to be unable to correct DNA damage. Cancer is a result of these mutations which interfere with oncogene and tumor suppression gene function and leads to this uncontrollable cell growth. Carcinogens are directly responsible for damaging DNA and promoting cancer. Free radicals are formed when our bodies are exposed to carcinogens. These free radicals damage cells and inhibit normal cell function.

If your family members; especially your parents and grandparents, have had cancer, it's obvious this gene mutation was passed on to you. But even so, this only means cancer forms quicker in these people than those without the family history of cancer. And as soon as your body is exposed to carcinogens, cancer begins to form. So, you can easily see how **avoiding poisons is the key to preventing and curing cancer. This is why all cancer patients should get serious about avoiding and eliminating poisons.**

Yep, that's what your doctor explained to you didn't he! No he didn't. Because he would lose a lot of money by telling you this. Poisons caused your cancer. And no doctor is going to tell you that, beyond mentioning cigarettes and alcohol, because the doctor knows that if you stop poisoning yourself, your cancer is going to fade away! So doctors have all these ways to "treat" your cancer and the symptoms that come with cancer. But no doctor is ever going to cure you of cancer or anything. You might want to explain to yourself WHY you think doctors COULD cure you, when no doctor has ever studied cures in medical school. As a matter of fact, and I do mean fact, doctors don't even practice medicine nowadays. But is all this about doctors going to cure you? Answer – NO!

What this talk about doctors is for, is to adjust your attitude that made you sick in the first place. And if you don't get your attitude adjusted to the realities of science and facts, then you only need to make sure your funeral coverage is paid up to date. And even IF doctors told you the cure for cancer, as I am going to do, they still couldn't cure you. And neither can I! But I know someone who CAN cure you. And it's the same person that made you sick in the first place.........YOU! Yes YOU are the one who can cure YOU.

YOU can learn to face the fact that poisons are NOT safe, no matter how often the FDA tells you they are certified "safe". Your parents told you poisons were bad for you. But you got all grown up and told everybody that you will do as you please, and that nobody is going to tell you what you CAN and can NOT eat! But you forgot to tell yourself that YOU are the one who is going to have the cancer those poisons cause.

So now it's time for YOU to clean your mess up and get to thinking outside that tiny bubble where you trusted your government and the corporations, all the way to cancer or some other chronic disease or diseases! Diseases are only chronic because you trust doctors with NO cures, to cure you! Pretty crazy, huh? I mean really; do you take your car to the grocery store to have a new muffler put on? No you don't! So why are you going to doctors for cures, when doctors have no cures and didn't even study cures in medical school!

Yep, the cure for cancer is easy to understand and do. But **you can't cure yourself as long as you are waiting on doctors and the medical profession to find the cures for cancer that already exists!** But plenty of you will walk for the cure for cancer, share cancer posts on Facebook in support of finding the cure for cancer that already exists. But the thing you never ever do is, share the cure for cancer with others!

In the City I live, there's all the big buzz about the new cancer "care" center they are building. And boy do doctors CARE about cancer. Yep, doctors care about keeping your cancer around so they can maximize their income off your suffering and pain, instead of telling you how to cure yourself of cancer. But there will never ever be a cancer CURE center in this town! Everything has to be threaded through money. Cures help people and save their lives. But cures take millions and billions of dollars of income from the medical profession. And that's why all cures are Dead On Arrival with doctors and the medical profession. And until cures start being taught in medical school, cures have no chance of being a part of the work of doctors and the medical profession.

So you have got to decide IF you want to live. And if you do, you can go ahead and cure yourself WHILE you still go to the doctor and follow all the quackery they have invented over the past 75 years, as doctors and the medical profession turned their backs on all cures and all medicine in the history of this planet.

Do you understand that 100% of the drugs your doctors prescribes you are removed naturally by your body? Your body begins to remove all drugs the moment they enter the body. That's why you have to keep taking them every day. But if doctors used real medicines, your body would put those real medicines to use in your body and only remove a small part of that real medicine. So am I saying to NOT take the drugs doctors prescribe you? NO I am not. What I am saying is that even the drugs your doctors prescribe you that do help you in some temporary way, are still poisons to your body that have to be completely removed. And to do that, your body uses up its own energy. Let me explain this a little more.

Your body only has so much energy. Your body needs energy to digest food, remove toxins, perform body metabolisms and repair damaged cells. You have got to learn to force your body to spend as much of its energy repairing damaged cells as you possibly can. Remember, cancer is caused by poisons damaging the nucleus of cells; which prevents the natural programmed death of cells. But if you stop stuffing those poisons down your throat, there won't be any poisons to cause cancer or any other chronic diseases!

I had a nice awakening to these scientific facts shortly after doctors told me I would be dead from chronic kidney disease by 2008 or 2009. I was talking to a nurse at the hospital and she mentioned that her husband had chronic kidney disease. I asked her what he was doing for his kidney disease. She said he was using ginger packs placed on his back next to his kidneys; and those ginger packs were soaking the poisons out of his kidneys. Now when she told me this, I got all excited and couldn't wait to start using the ginger packs to get those poisons out of me. But as I was trying to track down the ginger roots, I started thinking......now what if I don't put those poisons IN my body in the first place. Then there would be no need to soak them OUT of my kidneys! And that got my head to thinking a 100 miles an hour!

I started examining everything I ate and drank and everything my body comes in contact with; all the way from the food I eat, the water I drink and bathe in, and the personal hygiene items we all use, like soap, shampoo, conditioner and my underarm deodorants. And even though I have been an Organic Gardener for the past 30 years, still, I saturated my kidneys with so much poison in my drinks that they failed.

Lots of people said "Watch what you eat". But no one ever said "Watch what you DRINK" or "Watch what you shower in". And not doing that is what took out my kidneys after having arthritis, bleeding gums, intestinal bleeding and acid reflux for 20 years. Not to mention all the headaches I had all my life, like anybody else. I cured myself of all that and more.

As a matter of fact, I cured myself of every chronic disease and medical condition I had, by doing what I am going to be telling you in the chapters called Poisons in Your Water, Poisons in Your Drinks and Poisons in Your Food. But when it comes to a disease like cancer, you need to look beyond your food, drinks, water and hygiene items to stop exposing your body to poisons.

There are so many poisons and so many ways to become exposed to those poisons. That exposure can come in your work, play or other normal activities we all participate in. It can be the toxic foods all schools serve children, your garden supplies like pesticides, fungicides and fertilizers. Or working in a manufacturing plant, or food or drink corporations where they make these poisons that saturate the entire food and drinks supplies.

The constant principle that you MUST learn and understand, is that poisons cause ALL disease, except for the 20% caused by germs and viruses. And that by eliminating the poisons that caused the cancer in the first place, will cause the cancer to naturally fade away. This is the proven science that cures you. And this same proven science is the cure for every disease known to man. Without the poisons, there can be no disease. There can be NO cancer. But when most people hear these proven facts of science, they claim that they haven't been exposed to any real poisons. And that is where I have to point out the pride crushing facts about what a fool you really are. And I don't mean that in a mean way.

I rode the ship of fools until just a few years ago. So I don't have much room to talk. But I have abandoned the ship of fools through proven science which no doctor is willing to tell you. When I had bladder stones during the mid 90's, it is science that dictates that magnesium dissolves calcium and that bladder stones (and kidney stones and bone spurs) are formed by particles of calcium combining with toxins to form bladder and kidney stones. So I took magnesium oxide tablets and stopped my 4th bladder stone attack within an hour of it beginning, and have not had a bladder stone attack since then, 1996; which is 16 years as of now.

I could have learned all this BEFORE my 4th bladder stone attack. But I didn't. And that ignorance caused me a lot of pain and money! Doctors said there was no cure for bladder stones either. And when I called them to tell them I would pay all the UN-necessary tests and hospital bills if they would tell me the cure for bladder stones, what I got was threats. They threatened to call the Police and have me arrested if I didn't stop asking for the cure. They even called me the devil. I told them "OK, I'm the devil and you're calling the Police to have me arrested. But could you give me the cure for bladder stones?" But this only made them more irate!

This was after my 3rd bladder stone attack. And when the 4th one came, I was not going to consider the $1000+ ER bill and no cure I already got from them. And I sure the heck wasn't going to ask a damn doctor for a cure again and get called the devil and threatened with being arrested for it! So I took 2 250mg magnesium oxide tablets 30 minutes into my 4th bladder stone attack. And within an hour, the attack subsided and faded away. And that was THE END of bladder stone attacks in my life. Science works, and keeps on working!

When it comes to curing cancer, at first you might think that curing cancer is a whole lot harder than curing chronic kidney disease. And you would be wrong by a long shot. Everyone who gets chronic kidney disease, dies from it. A rare rare few get transplants that spare their lives. But since that transplanted kidney goes into that same person that already poisoned their kidneys into failure, they do the same thing to the new, healthy, transplanted kidney.

Without a lifestyle and diet change, no cure is possible. You have to choose whether you want to live OR you want to keep eating at restaurants, swigging sodas, eating red meat, cooking with the microwave, soaking your body with chlorine and filling your lungs with chlorine gas in the shower and a host of other bad habits that lead to sickness and a sure death, with no hope for anything better for you. It's very rare when it's just one poison that causes your chronic disease. It's the overloading of poisons that create sickness in your body. Let me give you a rundown of the huge amounts of poisons we all consume without any thought. Let's run through a day in most people's lives and stop to talk about it, every time your body is being poisoned. But before we do that, I need to cover just a few more things. You will see how this all fits together once you are finished reading this chapter and into the next chapter.

It's doing the things in the Chapters about Poisons in your food, drinks and water that ARE the cure for cancer, and the cure for any disease that ails or afflicts you. These chapters contain the information you will use on a daily basis as you learn to recognize poisons in order to avoid them. What I am doing now, is telling you the other things you need to know in order to make cures a reality for you, and in your life.

Cures are not a part of your life. You have always depended on doctors to fix the damage you do to your own body by ignoring science. That science has manifested itself as disease in your body. What I am teaching you is how to cause cures to manifest themselves in your body. And the first question you might have is "how is my body going to heal itself?" or "Can my body really heal itself of cancer?" The answer is YES! You already have the proof of that. But what am I talking about?

You have cut your finger before, right? You still have that cut? Well! I guess your body CAN heal itself. But even though all cuts you have ever had have healed and gone away, you didn't even know to put Vitamin E on those cuts to make them heal 3 times as fast and fade the scars much faster. But that science was always there, even when you had never heard of that. And the science to cure your cancer exists now, and has existed all along. But the cure for cancer and the cure for every disease has gained a vicious added element. So what use to cure cancer will no longer cure cancer. And that element is the saturation of addicting, poisons (drugs, chemicals, toxins) that corporations put in all their products. And the leading poison is high fructose corn syrup.

There is no worse disease causing substance than high fructose corn syrup. It's in everything. And when I say everything, I MEAN....everything. It's in your bread and everything sweet. And it's the main ingredient in countless Bar-BQ sauces, ketchups, salad dressings and things like that. And you have one choice of each of those items that are not saturated with HFCS. The worst things you can put in your body are soda pops and fruit juices. I explain this in the Chapters about Poisons in your food, drinks and water. I also explain how you are fooled by lying labels and catch phrases that never mean what they say, and the gimmicks of labeling products "low fat", "low sodium", "reduced calories", "All Natural" and other complete nonsense corporations use to trick you into continuing buying their poison saturated products, under the guise of being healthy.

Earlier, I told you we would take a look into a typical person's day and stop to talk about the poisons you come in contact with during normal daily activities. Let's do that right now...........

OK.......you just got a good night's sleep. The alarm clock goes off. You hit the snooze button, and get up 10 minutes later when the snooze goes off. Time to hit the bathroom for a shit, shower and shave or a wee wee! Ahh, you get into the shower and it hits you....that warm water all over your body making you feel good and stimulating you to wake on up. But what else is going on?

You are soaking your entire body, filling and soaking every pore on your body with deadly chlorine. Yea, chlorine is deadly. Hitler used it to murder millions of people in WW II. Yea, it's no secret. But you have kept this scientific fact out of your mind and thinking. It's time to wake up. That chlorine kills the oxygen in every cell it comes into contact with and also kills the oils in your skin and scalp. Now why would you have dandruff (dry scalp) by soaking your entire head and body with oxygen killing chlorine!

And you stand there in the shower playing Nazi against yourself; breathing in that hot water vapor with all that chlorine gas mixed in it! Gee......I can't figure out why that happens..........unless......unless... yea, I hope you guessed it........unless you include proven science in your thinking. Then you won't soak your entire body in chlorine and fluoride WHILE gassing yourselves with chlorine gas. But wait, you just got up to start your day, and that's just the shower.

So you get out of the shower and dry off with a chemically treated bath towel. Then soak your underarms with poisonous aluminum-zirconium or some other aluminum compound you can't pronounce. That harms your lymph nodes; which are your back up immune system. So, am I telling you to stop taking a shower and using underarm deodorants? NO. Read the Chapter titled Poisons in Your Water, and you'll know the solutions to these problems.

Then after saturating your body and lungs with deadly chlorine, you soak your underarms with toxic poisons and go to the table to have your breakfast. You sit down to eat some eggs, bacon, toast and coffee maybe. But what is that crap you are eating? All of it is acidic. That white bread toast is all poison. Your bacon and eggs have some nutritional value, but are soaked in chemicals from the feed the chicken and hogs eat; not to mention how hogs eat their own feces. Any acidic substance you put in your body inhibits normal body metabolisms. And the coffee is acidic too. That milk and sugar you put in your coffee are acidic. The milk has growth hormones, anti-biotics and other drugs milk cows are routinely injected with. And the sugar is pure poison. Sugar is a drug, not a food substance. Same is true of white flour. They're all drugs. Sugar has the same effect on your brain as cocaine does. (More on this later) Now it's time to go to work.

Now, you know more about your work places than I do. So I want you to take the time to write this part of the book with all the work places you work in, and all the obvious dangers and exposures to chemicals, dust and other toxins in your work places. And add those to all the stuff I am telling you now. But while you're at work, you most likely will eat that sugary crap and drink pure poison drinks at your work place.

And add the poisons you consume when you eat out at a restaurant for lunch. There's no healthy food or drinks at restaurants. The game to addict you to their food is just as intense as what you get from corporations in the grocery store. Poisoning you is Right and Safe, because the government says so! And the corporations laugh all the way to the bank. And your doctors follow behind them in squeezing as much money out of you, for the consequences of what the corporations caused in the first place. What a heinous racket! Then it's time to go home and eat supper.

Most people eat a pretty good supper. But most people have red meat and potatoes and tea. Pretty good eating, huh? Nope, not really. Once again you have the growth hormones, anti-biotics and all the other drugs beef cattle are injected with. And the poison soaked dead food they are fed. And you are eating their dead flesh! Oh well, those potatoes are pretty good for you, as long as you peel the poison soaked skin off of them, or at least scrub them with a steel brush! Then you boil them to leech out most of the nutrients. Then pour that water down the drain. The tea helps fight cancer and the lemon slice too. Then the sugar in the tea is still pure poison.

Now it's time to go brush your teeth again and soak your mouth with a host of chemicals. And maybe through the day, I took an antacid, Aleve or Tylenol. And I have a prescription or two I have to take. And all of it is poisons that your body has to remove. And that takes energy. And now you're off to bed, to start this cycle over again.

Now add all those poisons up, and you'll have no problem seeing WHY you have cancer or any other disease! And I didn't even count any snacks, cigarettes, alcohol or recreational drugs lots of people consume.

Now an extremely important thing you should do is use an inexpensive, common substance. It's almost silly what this substance is. It reverses the acidic condition that allowed your cancer to survive and thrive in your body. Cancer can NOT, I repeat, can NOT, live in an alkaline environment. And this common item is none other than baking soda, sodium bicarbonate; also called meetha soda. Cancer cells are also more acidic than the cells around the cancer.

Baking soda is pH 14, and when mixed with water makes the entire glass of water become a pH of 8.0-8-5. It can be more if you use a carbon water filter, and slightly higher if you use an osmosis system or fluoride filter. Merely mixing ¼ tea spoon in 6-8 ounces of water and drinking twice daily, before bed and when you awake, will serve as the foundation for your near certain cure.

And don't be fooled by the medical profession. They use sodium bicarbonate to keep chemotherapy patients from dying from the toxicity of their chemical drugs; and for clinical acidosis in patients. It's a vile story about why they stick with their dangerous expensive chemicals in spite of knowing safe, inexpensive natural medicinal solutions. It's all about greed, and greed with no thought of what is good for you, the patient! You would be well served to find a book by Dr. Mark Sircus tilted simply "Sodium Bicarbonate – Full Medical Review", 2nd edition; a book I only recently found out about. Dr. Sircus also has 2 books about curing cancer.

The near miraculous effects of sodium bicarbonate are explained in Dr. Sircus' book. Baking soda will relieve heartburn instantly. It also cures metabolic acidosis of your kidneys which causes almost all chronic kidney disease; and gets you well on your way to curing yourself of CKD. You can even brush your teeth with it.

Just wet your toothbrush. Shake it off once or twice. Then dip it in a box of baking soda to cover your brush with baking soda. Then brush and slosh the liquid around in your mouth a bit. This will neutralize the acid on your teeth and gums, and stop most tooth pain and lessen the severity of sensitivity to heat and cold. Wherever you need to kill fungus or neutralize an acidic substance, remember to call baking soda to the rescue!

There are so many things baking soda is good for. Some of its uses are that it absorbs radiation, alkalizes the body, absorbs heavy metal, treats colds and the flu, treats insect bites and itchy skin, soothes your feet and is a non-toxic deodorant. You can also use it to clean many things like dishes, floors, furniture, shower curtains, baby clothes and cloth diapers, cars, batteries, combs and brushes, and to clean the dirt and residue off fresh produce; as well as clean your bath tub, tile and sinks. Baking soda can also be used as a facial scrub and body exfoliant, to freshen linens, deodorize stinky feet and make a bath soak.

Although all of those uses are great, the lifesaving value of baking soda is the most important. It absorbs radiation, in case of a nuclear attack or exposure such as chemotherapy and radiation. Doctors and hospitals use baking soda to keep cancer patients from dying from radiation and chemotherapy.

And baking soda reverses the acidic state of your body that made it possible for you to develop chronic disease. So make sure you keep plenty of baking soda around. And make sure to drink 1/2 teaspoon baking soda with 4-6 ounces of water at least 2x daily, as the start and foundation of curing every disease you have and preventing disease from developing in the first place.

As we go to the next chapter to begin learning the things you have to know to recognize, reduce and eliminate disease causing poisons, remember that unless you believe you CAN be cured, it's never going to happen. I do NOT mean mind over matter or something stupid. I mean, that cures are not a part of your thinking, much less your life. In this country we have faith in our doctors that there ARE no cures for any diseases.

But because of people like me that know there are cures for every disease, and have cured ourselves of what doctors call "incurable" diseases, we're gonna tell you the Truth about the cures, and do everything we can to get this information to you. And hope that cures return to being a part of lives, communities and countries for the Protection, Welfare and Benefit of The People. But do NOT pretend that the helpless state of this country's sick care, health care system, is of The People, by The People or For The People.

The Cure For Cancer

2 - Let's Get You Started on Getting Rid of Your Cancer

This is where you start learning the things that will directly affect your cancer and train your body to heal itself. Still, there are no gimmicks. We are learning how to use science to heal our bodies, and how to speed that healing as much as we possibly can. You will need to use Chapters 3, 4 and 5 as your daily guide in getting rid of the saturation of poisons in your food, drinks and water supplies. But what I have told you so far is about attitude, state of mind; awakening to the fact that there IS a cure and you CAN be cured. You are going to cure yourself. And if you fall short, the least you will do is significantly improve your health and learn how to maintain that great improvement in your health.

I am not claiming to be some omnipotent, know it all. So there are so many different sets of circumstances in all the different people's lives. The one thing that does NOT change is science and its Laws of Physics. And that's why, if you do what this book says, you will certainly get the results stated. And for the skeptics and nay sayers, I can only quote My Cousin Vinny if you wanna claim these Laws of Science do NOT work for you........and that's "Are we supposed to believe that the Laws of Physics cease to exist at your house!" So do the things in this book WHILE you still go along with your doctors; except for the parts about Death and dying and there's no cure.

One of the major things you have to do, is start drinking lots of pure filtered water. That's why the Chapter called Poisons in Your Water begins the information you have to know to cure yourself. Your body is 80% water. And it ain't 80% water-chlorine and fluoride. So your body has to work to remove 100% of the chlorine and fluoride in your water. Drink 1 ounce of water for every 2 pounds of body weight. And try to use pH drops to raise the alkalinity of your drinking water. You can get pH drops on Ebay. One side effect of the highly alkaline water will be weight loss. As the highly alkaline water neutralizes acid in your body, your kidneys will remove all that water it retained to dilute that acid, as a natural defense to that acid. That is how you lose the weight.

Your water needs to be filtered. A carbon water filter only filters out about 90% of the chlorine and nothing else. So that's why you need a fluoride water filter at least. A reverse osmosis filter system is better and filters all your water in your home. Using either of these water filters takes all the taste out of your water that you taste in tap water. The chemicals are bitter and acidic. So by removing chlorine and fluoride, the bitter acidic taste is gone. And your water is alkaline. And to increase the alkalinity of your water, add pH drops to your drinking water every day. This raises the pH to around 7.5-8.0 and above.

Flushing your kidneys with this highly alkaline water will neutralize acid and slowly transform your body's acidic state back into the normal

alkaline state your body is supposed to be in. Your body became acidic over time as you consumed more and more animal products, sugar and chlorinated water. And the highly alkaline water reverses that disease ripe acidic environment inside your body. Chlorine destroys the oxygen in every cell it comes into contact with and kills the beneficial bacteria in your stomach and intestines. And your intestines are the central part of your immune system! Without your body being in this acidic state from consuming chlorinated water and animal products, your cancer would never have become a chronic disease.

You have to remember that your body is always making cancer cells. But when you overload your body and immune system with too many poisons for an extended period of time, your body is unable to remove cancer cells and other toxins as fast as they form. So they begin to gather in places in the body.

As cancer cells gather in your body, they will begin to cling to tissue and organs and begin to form blood vessels. This allows cancer cells to be carried to almost any place in your body. You've heard the doctors tell you this by saying "The cancer is spreading." So what can you do to arrest your cancer and send it into permanent remission, aka "cure"?

Start taking Vitamin C, Fish or Flax seed oil and magnesium. Why? Because your diet is deficient in all of these. Why are Vitamin C, Fish or Flax seed oil and magnesium so important?

First of all, this savage red meat "American diet" is insane to begin with. Men don't have the teeth for chewing meat. You need sharp fangs to cut and chew meat. We humans don't have sharp fangs. We are supposed to be on a fish diet, not this savage red meat diet. The fish oil has the Omega-3 that your body must have or you develop diseases like arthritis, Alzheimer's, Parkinson's, heart disease and cancer. Flax seed oil is a vegetable source of Omega-3.

You need about 1000mg of Fish or Flax seed oil daily to maintain your health and prevent disease. You need 3-4 times that amount while you are sick. And try to eat fish as often as possible. Eat fish types that have scales like Cod, Tilapia, Salmon and Tuna. Catfish does NOT have scales.

Next, you need lots of Vitamin C. Why? Because Vitamin C is a common and readily available anti-oxidant. Anti-oxidants are the substances that remove toxins from your body. Your body does NOT store Vitamin C. So it is up to you to make sure you give your body a steady supply of Vitamin C. You should take at least 5000mg of Vitamin C daily if you have cancer. Taking more is better. Up to 10,000mg daily is what you should try to take. But increase your dose of daily Vitamin C gradually until you are at that level dosage.

You should also consider taking other anti-oxidants like Selenium, Beta-Carotene (Vitamin A), Vitamin E and other lesser known anti-oxidants. Vitamin

E is a great way to speed repair to damaged cells both inside and out. You can find more information about most of these food substances in Chapter 6.

But why do you have to take the magnesium? For one, magnesium is needed to perform over 300 body metabolisms. Without sufficient magnesium, these body functions don't occur. Add to that, the certain acidic state of your body which has already habitually inhibited all body metabolisms, and you have a state of death settling into your body. And can you tell me where you are getting enough magnesium in your diet? No you can't. So take the magnesium supplements; at least 250-400mg twice daily if you are sick; 250-400mg most days to maintain your health and prevent disease. I already told you that unless you take magnesium vitamins, you are bound to form bladder or kidney stones and/or bone spurs. And correcting these major nutrient deficiencies in your diet will go a long way in your efforts to improve your health as you work toward your goal of being cured.

Once you do what I've told you so far, you will be on your way to reversing that acidic, disease ripe state of your body, begin to lose weight, begin to feel better almost every day, and notice that your body is recovering within 3-4 weeks. That improvement will depend on how well you conform your food, drinks and water to what is told in Chapters 3, 4 and 5 and correct these MAJOR diet deficiencies. Let's take a look at a commonly known beverage that leads the way to many diseases. These poisons are bad for you in every way.

Now, a good example of how bad all those poisons are, is when you drink a soda pop. People fool themselves by thinking that soda pop gives them a welcome energy boost! But it's no energy boost! What really happens is this: You begin drinking that high fructose corn syrup soaked soda in liquid form with that DNA altering sodium benzoate and that 3.0 acidic carbonated water. And your body goes into instant shock as it tries to defend itself against all that poison. This instant elevated activity the body goes into to remove these poisons is what we falsely tell ourselves is a harmless, healthy energy boost. And it takes your body up to 6 hours to remove the poisons in a 12 ounce soda pop. That cripples your immune system. And by drinking a 12 ounce soda every 6 hours, you in effect, nullify your immune system. And this is just one example of what you will learn in Chapters 3, 4 and 5.

Fasting - Another major thing you can do to speed your healing is to fast. It is not necessary to fast for days. By simply eating your last meal around 6 PM, then not eating again until between 6 and 10 AM the next day, will do a lot for you; especially if you make it a habit. Fasting was the foundation of the medical practices of Hippocrates, the Father of Medicine. What fasting does is to relieve the body of the most energy consuming bodily task of digesting food. Once your body ceases to digest food, your body then uses that energy to repair damaged cells in our bodies. And when you are sick, your body needs to use as much energy as possible to repair damaged cells and remove toxins. And the less poisons you put into your body, the more energy your body has to use to remove those toxins.

Your body only has so much energy. It uses most of its energy to digest food. It uses the rest of its energy to remove toxins and repair damaged cells. So you have to learn how to make your body use more and more of its energy to repair damaged cells to heal and cure you. The easiest way to do that is to fast as often as possible and cut down on the amount of food you eat. Using chapters 3, 4 and 5 to reduce the amount of poisons you consume in your food, drinks and water will relieve your body of having to use so much energy to remove toxins from your body. Doing this and fasting allows your body to use most of its energy to repair damaged cells, which eventually results in you being cured.

No matter how long you can manage to fast, remember to drink plenty of pure water. If you go more than 2 or 3 days without food, don't hesitate to eat a bite of fruit or raw vegetables. Stuff like that aids in your healing and doesn't take much energy to digest.

But why hasn't your doctor told you to do this? Your doctors are the ones who swore an Oath to Hippocrates when they became "doctors". But they're not telling you about the main part and foundation of the Medical Practices of Hippocrates, the Father of Medicine. I have never sworn an Oath to Hippocrates. But I'm the one telling you "Do what the Father of Medicine did".

Now, with 133,000,000 Americans who have at least one chronic disease, is that what you call the result of the best health care system in the world? Yes you do! But it's complete nonsense. Each of those 133,000,000 Americans represents a failure of this country's medical profession. Even with 10,000,000 Americans with chronic disease, we should have declared a national emergency.

But with 133,000,000 Americans with at least one chronic disease, we not only haven't declared a national emergency, we continue to declare that we have the best health care on the planet! If every single person had at least one chronic disease, they would still tell you that; and you would still believe them! I don't know of any greater incompetence in any profession or line of work than this country's medical profession and health care system.

When I got those statistics above from the Center for Disease Control web site, http://www.cdc.gov/chronicdisease/overview/index.htm I noticed their web site also talked about what causes these chronic diseases. But guess what they did NOT mention in that information? Not one word about poisons in your food, drinks and water supplies. The closest they came was naming cigarettes or alcohol as a cause of lung cancer or liver disease. Whoop dee

Do! But it's the same thing at the doctor's office! Rarely does a doctor tell you what caused your chronic disease. I have asked almost everyone I have talked to, if their doctor has ever told them what caused their chronic disease. I never get any specific answers; just vague generalizations!

Now that's what you should be getting from rank amateurs, but NOT from professionals! A professional is assumed to be an expert in their field or occupation. But how can you call the medical profession that has failed to cure the diseases of over 133,000,000 people at this very moment, "experts"! Face reality as it is. With over 133,000,000 known cases of complete failure by this country's doctors and medical profession, it's well past time to try something new. You know.....something that does NOT have 133,000,000 known failures at any given moment!

People prefer to eat as much poisons as they choose and never think about what they're doing. They think they can run to the doctor and the doctor will save them from the consequences of their own actions. But what they end up with is one lifelong disease after another, and a pile of prescriptions to take every day. You trust your food supply to be safe. You trust your drinks to be safe. You trust your water supplies to be safe. I've got some advice for you.......Stop trusting your food, drinks and water suppliers. What fluoride has to do with safe drinking water is a scam that continues as I write. Don't trust your water company and prove it by getting a water filter to protect yourself. You can afford a water filter. But you can't afford the medical bills that the chlorine and fluoride will burden you with. Again, it costs about $30-40 a year to prevent brittle bones, bladder cancer and a ravaged immune system, compared to the thousands to tens of thousands of $$$$$ in medical bills for treating the diseases caused by the chlorine and fluoride. You can afford the preventions, but not the treatments.

And stop trusting your food, drinks and water suppliers. I am not talking about the grocery stores either! The grocery store puts the garbage on the shelves that you buy again and again. If you didn't buy those poison soaked products, they would stop buying those products from their suppliers. Grocery stores stock their shelves with products that sell the fastest. And guess what? For the most part, the healthiest products are the cheapest. If only you were lucky enough to only be able to afford dry beans and brown rice!!!! There are rare few exceptions. The most significant is with bread.

White bread is cheap, but has little to no real nutritional value; whereas whole wheat bread costs 3 times as much, but is highly nutritious. But since bread is a diet staple, you count on eating bread regularly. So it needs to be healthy and nutritious. Otherwise, you get the diseases and conditions white flour and bread cause, starting with chronic diarrhea and intestinal bleeding. You can afford the cure, prevention. But you can't

afford the treatments. The choice is yours to make. Just remember that it is you that has to make the changes.

One other major help in speeding you toward your cure is drinking Sage and/or Lemon Balm tea. Sage was a cure all to Indians, Still is. And Lemon Balm was a cure all to the Egyptians. I had a great experience drinking Lemon Balm tea when my kidneys failed. It sent healing warmth into every part of my insides it came into contact with. It was the only bright spot in the days of my worst nightmare. I know it works; same as Sage. One thing is that they have good amounts of anti-oxidants. You can find more information on Sage and Lemon Balm at the end of this book; in Chapter 6.

You also have to understand that you need to eat as healthy a diet and drinks as you can. I mean, why drink a soda or fruit juice when you could drink something that your body doesn't have to work so hard to remove. You could drink fruit smoothies made with raw fruits. That would be almost 100% good for your body. Those live fruits and vegetables have enzymes that pump life into your body.

And your body doesn't work to remove that live produce. Your body uses most of that live produce. And if you juice that produce, it's easier for your body to digest than solid food. So it takes far less energy to digest that produce if you run them through a good juice making machine. But even if you don't juice or don't do it often, you can still try to eat as much raw fruits and vegetables as you possibly can.

As a matter of fact, **if you just get those water filters and just follow what I call The Perfect Diet, you can cure yourself or significantly improve your health without having to learn how to read food labels and avoid the masses of products that are saturated with poisons; most of which we pretend are food.** So what do I mean by The Perfect Diet? The Perfect Diet is the best diet to be on. But since it is a far cry from the "American diet", you may do best by using Chapters 4 & 5 to clean up your current diet that caused your diseases in the first place.

The Perfect Diet….

What do I mean by The Perfect Diet? If I could eat the most healthy diet of food and drinks, what would that diet consist of? Right off you would say eat fresh fruits and vegetables ONLY and drink pure water The problem you would have is that there are poisons inside all produce in this country. So you would have to buy all Organic; which is not possible without restricting your diet even further. You could grow all the produce yourself, or hire someone to do it for you, if you can afford to. So, the perfect diet is not practical in this country and the life styles we live in this country.

You could grow all your own food organically and drink pure water. But as soon as you are forced to send your children to school, they'll gag them with poison saturated food. But the Perfect Diet would be to grow all your food organically and drink pure water. You can grow peaches, figs, apples, grapes, Kiwi, Strawberries and all kinds of fruits to go along with your organic vegetables. Stick to drinking pure water, and you're on the Perfect Diet! But since we all know how impractical this is, we have to present an idea or ideas that are achievable for most people. So how do we come close to having the Perfect Diet, living in this country?

The obvious is just buy produce from the grocery store and wash it extra good, and make as much of that produce as you can, Organic produce. Then buy Organic 2% milk. Eat lots and lots of brown rice. Drink Lipton tea sweetened with Stevia. Buy only whole fish or fillets. No breading. Bake your own whole grain breads and don't add the sick crap to them, like vegetable oils, margarine, white flour and white granulated sugar. Buy frozen produce when fresh is not available. Never buy canned. And use raw honey anywhere you want and as much as you want. Drink lots of pure Noni, Goji and Mangosteen juice or Goji berries. Add dried fruits and nuts to your diet. And even adding all these things beyond the ultimate Perfect Diet, you still have a near perfect diet.

And that's The Perfect Diet! You will want to read on and use Chapters 4 & 5 as a guide from now on to avoid those poisons that saturate our entire food and drinks supplies. And keep the principles in mind at all times that I just discussed in this chapter, and Chapter 1, while you change to The Perfect Diet or choose to clean up your current diet by using Chapters 4 and 5 as your guide. Your body is 80% water. Drinking 1 ounce of water per 2 pounds of body weight daily helps clean out your body and flush large amounts of toxins out through your urine.

So let's get on to the rest of the information you need to guide you, as you **switch from your present "Doctor care Sick Care" to taking charge of your own health and helping yourself 24 hours a day, on your way to much better health and very likely curing yourself!**

So I begin with **Poisons in Your Water.**

The Cure For Cancer

3 -Poisons in Your Water

It is very important that I talk to you about the poisons in your water first. The first city to provide chlorinated water in the US was Jersey City in 1908. At least 70% of the US population gets their water from systems relying on chlorine; although 90% of the water systems in the US rely on chlorination in one form or the other. Chlorine was first used in water supplies to stop typhoid. Researchers claim this actually worked, and have presented proof that chlorine kills other water borne diseases. I don't doubt any of this. As a matter of fact, if it wasn't for the chlorine in your water you would get sick shortly after drinking water in city water systems.

So I agree that the chlorine needs to be in the water to kill germs. But guess what? Chlorine kills bacteria. Oh, you already knew that! LOL But what rare few ever realize is that chlorine keeps right on being itself and kills bacteria once it's inside your body. And that is what no one is talking about. Your water supplier sure doesn't want to talk about it either.

I called our water supplier called CW&L. The Manager of CW&L certainly admitted to the chlorine and fluoride they put in our water. But he refused to agree to warn the Public about the dangers and adverse consequences of drinking and showering in their chlorinated water. I told him point blank "You need to take the fluoride out of the water. It should never have been put in our water." As he pretended to defend his position in favor of the poisons, he pointed out how beneficial fluoride is in preventing a few cavities. What he didn't want to talk about is what fluoride has to do with safe drinking water or the many cases of brittle bones, chromosome damage and other conditions known to be caused by fluoride ingestion.

The fluoride in drinking water has absolutely no benefit beyond this claim about preventing cavities. But hey, we could add vitamin C to the water. It's good for you. Or add other things that are good for us. That is, if you don't care about clean water! Whoops! You mean CW&L has lost touch with reality and no longer realizes that our water supply is NOT the place to be adding chemicals or anything else.

Water is H2O, NOT H2O+chlorine+fluoride! I want WATER, H2O! But I can't get it. So I gotta give it to myself by getting a fluoride water filter. It would be so easy IF CW&L would stop being CWL&Dental and start being CW&L again! But they refuse. So I gotta keep using a fluoride water filter. No problem, except for the $110 to buy a fluoride water filter.

But even though chlorine and fluoride cause a host of diseases, the most significant damage that immediately affects everyone who drinks it is how chlorine kills the beneficial bacteria in your stomach and intestines. Remember, I already pointed out that chlorine is in your water to kill bacteria!

And *chlorine keeps right on killing bacteria once it's inside your body!* Is this good? NO. That beneficial bacteria in your stomach and intestines is required to sustain your life. As these bacteria, flora, are killed your body digests less of your food. This issue is so important that I want you to read some technical facts about this bacteria, gut flora. So I am including what Wikipedia says about this, even though most of you can just SEARCH Wikipedia for "gut flora". Here's exactly what Wikipedia states:

Gut flora consists of microorganisms that live in the digestive tracts of animals and is the largest reservoir of human flora. Gut (the adjective) is synonymous with intestinal, and flora with microbiota and micro flora.

The human body, consisting of about 100 trillion cells, carries about ten times as many microorganisms in the intestines. The metabolic activities performed by these bacteria resemble those of an organ, leading some to liken gut bacteria to a "forgotten" organ. It is estimated that these gut flora have around 100 times as many genes in aggregate as there are in the human genome.

Bacteria make up most of the flora in the colon and up to 60% of the dry mass of feces. Somewhere between 300 and 1000 different species live in the gut, with most estimates at about 500. However, it is probable that 99% of the bacteria come from about 30 or 40 species. Fungi and protozoa also make up a part of the gut flora, but little is known about their activities.

Research suggests that the relationship between gut flora and humans is not merely commensal (a non-harmful coexistence), but rather a symbiotic relationship. Though people can survive without gut flora, the microorganisms perform a host of useful functions, such as fermenting unused energy substrates, training the immune system, preventing growth of harmful, pathogenic bacteria, regulating the development of the gut, producing vitamins for the host (such as biotin and vitamin K), and producing hormones to direct the host to store fats. However, in certain conditions, some species are thought to be capable of causing disease by producing infection or increasing cancer risk for the host.

Now that you have some in depth information about the bacteria, flora, in your stomach and intestines and its tremendous importance, now I'll tell you how killing this bacteria, by drinking chlorinated water, affects you and your health. The most common condition affects how much you eat. Almost all of us drink chlorinated water our entire childhood lives. After 18 years of doing this you have significantly reduced the amount of good bacteria in your stomach and intestines. As a result, you eat a good meal, but you are hungry again within an hour and a half to two hours later. Why? Because you are mistaking the barren feeling in your stomach as hunger pains. So you eat food to feel something in your stomach.

Eating sugary foods, drinking sugary drinks and eating white flour aggravates and burns your stomach and intestines making this empty barren feeling even worse! Then heartburn begins as a further sign of this damage to your stomach and intestines. Then your intestines begin to bleed and you bleed out your bunghole, or rectum for you technically minded people. Your doctor calls this bleeding ulcers, but can't really do a thing for you; although doctors do trick people into having surgery to correct this. Uh, cough, gag, stumble, puke! But is there any condition that doctors do NOT claim you need surgery for?!? Yes you need surgery so doctors can make big bucks off your disease and suffering.

But for you to be cured of bleeding ulcers, you're gonna need to learn what I am telling you. I wish I could charge a small percentage of the huge amounts of money the information in this book saves you, compared to what the medical industry charges you to never cure you, but treat and drug your diseases and medical conditions. I could hire you as my servants! LOL Sorry. I know how serious this is, but the helpless corrupt medical profession makes me laugh.

What can I do to replenish this good bacteria killed by chlorine? There are several things you can do. You can take probiotics. That's what I did. Believe me. I didn't know much of anything when I was learning the things I talk about in this book. So I used myself as a guinea pig to experiment and test these things to save my own life, or end up on dialysis by 2008 or dead by 2009 as the doctors insisted. I started taking probiotics. I started out just taking some Lactobacillus acidophilus and B. Lactis, also known as Acidophilus complex. But once I started taking Dr. Ohirra's Probiotics 12 Plus I started noticing some improvement. I wasn't hungry shortly after eating and my stomach felt much better.

I am still taking Dr. Ohirra's Probiotics from time to time and take the Acidophilus complex daily, usually more than once a day with meals. Buy the Acidophilus with the most active cultures. I use the one with 1 billion live organisms per capsule. Capsules are much easier to digest and therefore provide the greatest benefit compared to caplets or tablets. Acidophilus is the easiest pro-biotic to find. It's one of two bacteria usually found in yogurt. Probiotics with 10-12 different bacteria or more are a little harder to find, but provide the greatest health benefits; especially a natural probiotics product such as Dr. Ohhira's Probiotics.

Eating fresh, raw fruits and vegetables aid in the production of beneficial bacteria in your stomach and intestines too. The enzymes in raw fruits and vegetables are the key to this aid, and do so many other beneficial things to improve your health and heal your body. So eat as much fresh, raw fruits and vegetables as you can. There are lots of books explaining the endless health benefits of fresh fruits and vegetables, so I will not go into this in depth. Fresh fruits and vegetables provide generous amounts of fiber to protect your stomach and intestines, aid in digestion, nourish and heal damaged cells and promote regular bowel movements.

People whose diets are lacking in fresh fruits and vegetables and fiber rarely have bowel movements every day. Fact is, you should have a bowel movement not too long after each meal. Most of you will say that's crazy. No one has a bowel movement after each meal or most meals! But what I say to you is this...it's NOT crazy either. Want some proof?

Oki dokey people! Any of you ever have children? Ah ha! You only changing poopy diapers ONCE each day! I think NOT! When you are born and a baby, your stomach and intestines are healthy. You know, before you start killing your insides with chlorinated water, antibiotics, sugars and more. So you poop after each meal usually. But as you bombard your intestines with all these poisons, your body goes to work trying to protect itself against all these poisons. As a result, your intestines get coated with mucus.

Mucus looks like snot and boogers mixed together; which you see in your poop quite often. Once this mucus coats your intestines, your intestines have a harder and harder time of digesting and absorbing nutrients. In addition, you start developing pockets in your intestines which your poop begins to move into. Some people have 5-10 pounds of poop stuck in these pockets in your intestines; which stay in your intestines rotting for years, causing even more discomfort and health problems.

Doing a colon cleanse will do a lot in solving this problem. There are lots of different colon cleanses on the market. Most of them aren't very good. But I have tried a few of them. The best ones I have found are called Colonix and Almighty Cleanse. But here's a link you can go to and read about the top colon cleansers and make your own choice. www.detoxreviews.com If you do any internal cleanses, make sure you do a colon cleanse first. That way, if you did a liver cleanse, kidney cleanse or any other internal cleanse you won't cause yourself problems by overloading your intestines with poisons. So cleanse your colon, then do other cleanses to be safe and as effective as possible.

Although the cause of Elvis Presley's death was ruled as a heart attack, his doctors had treated Elvis for chronic constipation for over a decade before his death, and now believe Elvis's death was actually caused by chronic constipation. Elvis' autopsy revealed that Elvis' digestive system was a real mess when he died and that Elvis would've have lived longer if he had a colostomy. I know that doing a colon cleanse certainly helped me. The proof was how it made me feel better and lighter inside and by looking at my own poop when I was doing colon cleanses. I go by results, not the price of the product or the sales pitch and advertisements about the product.

I want to point out to you right now that it was necessary for me to talk about the poisons in your water first, before I talked about anything else for a very good reason. As you read this book there are many things I recommend that you put into your body. But these vitamins, herbs, foods and other items have to be digested properly. So the more beneficial bacteria you have in your stomach and intestines, the better you digest these items and thus, the more you benefit from taking them.

In some people these vitamins, herbs and foods may seem to do you very little good if the beneficial bacteria in your stomach and intestines is greatly depleted. So, for these vitamins, herbs and foods to do you more good and benefit you more greatly you will need to take probiotics as the first thing to do. Then you will get the greatest benefits from taking supplements, herbs and healthy foods in the most cost effective and efficient manner.

About the most important thing you can do about the poisons in your water is to get some type of water filter. You need one for your drinking and cooking water and one for your shower. Yes, you need a shower filter. But first let's look at the solution for needing a water filter. You can buy inexpensive faucet end carbon water filters. Years ago, we bought a Water Pik faucet end filter. It does a lot of good for about $20. You can buy easily replaceable carbon filter cartridges for about $5 each or a 4 pack for around $16. We got ours at Lowe's back in the 80's and used it till we got a cylinder shaped counter top carbon water filter from HSN. These filters are worth the money if that is all you can afford or care to invest at first. What you really need is a fluoride filter. A carbon filter only filters out about 90% of the chlorine, some dirt and other impurities, but not a speck of fluoride. Fluoride is a smaller particle and requires a better filter to eliminate it.

Fluoride filters – Fluoride filters are my filter of choice. Sure, I'd like to have a whole house osmosis filtration system, but the fluoride water filter we use is really great. The chlorine and fluoride give tap water a bitter taste which you get use to after drinking it that way for years. But I always do a little test to show people the difference between water and chlorinated, fluoridated water.

I take two identical glasses. Pour chlorinated, fluoridated water in one glass and pure water from our fluoride water filter in the other glass, and ask them to tell me if they can tell any difference and which one they like the best. 100% of the people so far always say the water that came from the fluoride water filter is the best and know which is which. I also ask them "What does the water from the fluoride filter taste like?" Their answer "Nothing" or "It doesn't have any taste". I tell them "Right, because it's WATER!"

When we first got our fluoride water filter, my wife and I would giggle every time after drinking some water. Hey, don't bash us! hehe We couldn't help it. Every drink of water going down our throats is pure and tasteless! Neither of us had ever had that experience. We felt highly privileged to be drinking water so pure. We even thought it was stupid that we felt that way about a water filter! Problem is, we are worse about it now than we were at the first. I love that pure water. You can drink all you want and it does absolutely no harm, and does so much good for your body and your health.

Having pure water from our fluoride water filter may have been the #1 factor in saving my life or at least sparing my life for years so far. Even doctors will tell you that your kidneys love water. And the fact that I was diagnosed with chronic kidney disease a few months earlier made pure water become the thing I began to consume the most. **You need one ounce of water for every two pounds of body weight daily.** For me that's around three quarts daily.

I never drank that much water in my life, and the older I got the less water I drank. Fortunately for me, the past 30 years I've been drinking filtered water. I sometimes think about how much chlorine I have NOT consumed and the internal damage that comes with drinking tap water. Your body has to filter out every bit of that chlorine and fluoride, and almost all of that work is handled by your kidneys. Once your kidneys get saturated with so much poison that they can't remove all of it from your body as quickly as you pour and stuff those poisons down your throat, your kidneys will begin to fail. I'll tell you how that happened to me in Chapter 8.

What about a shower filter? I believe a shower filter is at least as important as having a filter on your drinking and cooking water. I never thought about having a shower filter my whole life and honestly had never heard of such a thing. I didn't know anything about shower filters until after I bought one. Now, sometimes I get to thinking a shower filter is more important than a filter for drinking and cooking water; which bolsters my opinion that you need both and should see them both as necessities. The main reason I believe this is because **you soak up about ten times as much chlorine and fluoride in the shower as you generally do through drinking and cooking water.**

Water causes the pores in your skin to expand; which allows greater absorption into your body and bloodstream. After we got our shower filter I could tell right off that the water coming out of the shower filter no longer had that chemical chlorine smell. I even got a large glass of tap water to sniff in the shower; which I then sniffed the water coming out of the shower filter. The tap water had that familiar chlorine smell, and the filtered shower water had no smell. Then I just left it to hopefully do what I bought it for.

A few weeks later my wife and I both got a good surprise. We have had burning itchy places on our bodies over the years. We blamed cold weather, taking too many showers and maybe a few other things, but never got rid of those itchy red places. When I looked back soon after this, I realized while in the shower that those red itchy places were the exact places where the most shower water hits my body.

Our good surprise was that we no longer had those red itchy places just 3 weeks after installing our shower filter! I got on the INTERNET to SEARCH for something to explain our good surprise. As it turns out, the chlorine in tap water destroys the oils in your skin...and...and...YOUR HAIR! Got dandruff! I bet you do after burn drying your scalp with chlorinated water! I repeat...the chlorine in your shower water dries out your skin, scalp and hair by destroying the oils in your skin, scalp and hair!

Don't calm down yet! LOL Here's what could be the worst part... (I say this very sincerely and make the following comparison to save lives, and for this reason, the following should not offend anyone.) We all know Hitler used chlorine gas to murder millions of people. So, there's not a one of us who does not know how wrong this is, and should not be done to anyone. But guess what? Almost every one of you are doing the same thing to yourself, and doing it daily in most cases.

You got that hot chlorinated water steaming up the shower enclosure and that chlorinated steam goes right into your lungs and into your blood stream as fast as possible. Remember when I pointed out that YOU are the one who made YOU sick? Who told you chlorine gas was safe! Oh yeah...I forgot to mention that HUGE fact that the result of ingesting chlorine damages every cell it comes in contact with. Search the INTERNET to find information about all the various specific damage chlorine is known to do to your body. Check Wikipedia too.

Where do I buy probiotics, a carbon or fluoride water filter and a shower filter? I confess to buying them all off Ebay. Ha ha! You can also get some probiotics from Puritans Pride – www.puritans.com . And of course, there are lots of places on the INTERNET. We have bought from Puritan's Pride for almost 30 years. We were buying from Nutrition Headquarters who were later bought by Puritan's Pride. We buy vitamins, herbs, soap and other items from Puritans Pride too. We place an order every 2 or 3 months.

The shower filter we use is made by Crystal Quest. Search Ebay for KDF shower filter. Shower filters use a special carbon filter known as a KDF filter. This type shower filter uses a carbon filter which is designed for filtering hot water. If you run hot water through any carbon filter that is not specified as a KDF filter, the hot water will cause your carbon filter to dissolve. So make sure you purchase a KDF filter and don't be running hot water through any of the carbon or fluoride filters you use for your drinking and cooking water; which is connected to your kitchen faucet.

Beware that when we bought our first shower filter in early 2007, we couldn't find one at any store in this hub of commerce City of 55,000 people. Hard to believe, but it's true. And of course, SEARCH the INTERNET for the store of your choice if you don't care for Ebay.

As for a water filter for cooking and drinking water, I always recommend a disposable counter-top fluoride filter from Pure Water Essentials. This one at http://purewateressentials.com/ct-00145.html

It costs $100 plus shipping of around ten dollars. It lasts for years. Pure Water Essentials sells all types of water filters. So you can browse their site and find what's best for you. But I have recommended this filter to everyone so far.

What about bottled water? The simple answer is...don't be a fool! Buying bottled water is foolish and a waste of money, unless there are some odd circumstances I haven't thought of. If the gas company has fracked your water supply you could need bottled water. Fracked water will ruin your water filter in no time! Bottled water contains more than water. I looked and looked and looked for bottled WATER, but could only find bottled water with several other ingredients! The best bottled water I found was Ozarka. It has the fewest ingredients. You can get about ONE THOUSAND times as much filtered water by buying a counter top water filter than you get buying bottled water.

Some bottled water is just tap water in a bottle too. And your fluoride filtered water is pure. Bottled water never is. So your body has to filter out those added ingredients. I bought bottled water one time, and that was enough to convince me to never buy any more.

Remember, the information in this book is not only to prevent and cure disease...it can and will save you lots and lots of money. And that's the bottom line 'cause...whoops, don't want Stone Cold Steve Austin claiming I was using his catch phrase. So that's the bottom line 'cause...if I told you otherwise, I'd be lying.

4 -Poisons in Your Drinks

Now here's the subject that almost killed me and still shocks me and pisses me off sometimes…the poisons in our drinks. I have been an organic gardener since 1981, so I have eaten very healthy food all these years. I even trimmed the fat off all the meat I ate, to be safe. Sure I ate some bad foods. But it wasn't very often or very much. And even though I was the healthiest eater among family, friends and acquaintances, quite often people would say "Watch what you eat". "Oh I do" I would tell them, and it was the truth. I only had one cold/flu since 1981 and no serious illness for nearly two decades, so my health confirmed I was eating right. And guess what? I really was! But you know what no one EVER told me?

What I never told myself either? No one ever said "Watch what you DRINK". Oh how I wish with all my mind and body that someone would've told me that! Oh how I wish I had told myself that! But no one did, and I never did. I didn't tell anyone to watch what they drink either. But I was good at telling people "watch what you eat".

I know most of you are wondering what the blues blazes am I talking about! Don't feel bad about it. I felt like Columbus setting sail to sail off the edge of the earth and like Lewis and Clark westward explorations. I was heading into unknown territory! Why the very idea of thinking something bad about beloved companies who make Coke, Pepsi, Dr. Pepper, Ocean Spray, Gatorade, Welch's and the rest.

All their products are verified "safe" by the FDA. But what their products had done to my health compelled and convinced me to at least consider bad things about those products. At first I was lost as to figure out what blew out my kidneys. I tell the story in Chapter 7 about how I came to learn almost all the cures I have proven and learned about and what happened that forced me to face up to reality as it really is, about everything I was eating, drinking or coming into contact with.

When I began to learn the magnitude of how poisoned our drinks supply is, my incurable chronic kidney disease began to improve; instead of getting progressively worse and end in death. The only options doctors gave me was dialysis within 2 years and death likely shortly thereafter. I would need a kidney transplant at that point to avoid death. So I was determined to find out what caused my kidneys to fail, even though the doctors could never tell me. It was hypertension that blew my kidneys, but they couldn't tell me what caused my high blood pressure either. One doctor said it was probably salt. But none of my metabolic tests ever backed that up or even hinted to such a thing. So all I could do is wonder what caused this. I was lost as anyone could be and felt so helpless. But one day that all began to change.

As I began to pay attention to how I felt; examining, scrutinizing and analyzing how I felt all day long, I began to recognize a reoccurring bad sick feeling. I had been scrambling to find something to drink to replace the sugar soaked sweet tea I loved to guzzle down at every meal. So I got me some fruit juices. I got the ones that said they were made from concentrate. Gee. I'm about to drink some totally healthy fruit juice and not only that, it's concentrated fruit juice! Yippee. Roll out the success mat. I've got something healthy to drink, and lots of it. But then, here comes that mean a-hole, Mr. Reality and Mr. Facts to boot…and there goes my fruit juices! The problem is that I thought concentrate meant they boiled the fruit juice down to make a concentrated form of that juice.

I was wrong. The FDA guidelines for claiming something as concentrate basically means…packed with as much sugar or high fructose corn syrup as they choose to put in their products. I kept reading fruit juice cans and jars looking for any juice that was not made from concentrate. As I read the labels I keep noticing high fructose corn syrup in the ingredients. My wife and I kept throwing our hands up in disbelief about this. The reality is, that **once you start trying to eliminate high fructose corn syrup, the grocery store becomes a much smaller place.**

When I started looking for fruit juices without high fructose corn syrup, I was still chugging' down the cranberry juice. I was just blind to the facts. I had been drinking this most popular brand of cranberry juice and bragged about how healthy it was for me. Of course, I hadn't read the label either. Turns out it has more sugar declared on the label than your most popular brands of soda pops. I thought, no this can't be true. Something as good for you as cranberry juice and they packed it with poison. It made no sense. It couldn't be true. OR maybe I was just full of you know what. It rhymes with mit.

So I drank some cranberry juice and within 10 minutes I had that tense sick feeling again. I realized that I had that feeling every time I drank some cranberry juice after my kidneys failed. But it was so out of place and downright insane that something so good for you was really extremely bad for you. I had been drinking a quart a day almost every day for almost 3 years. All that time I thought I was so smart to be drinking cranberry juice almost every day. I never even stopped to think it might be bad for you. I tossed out the last of the cranberry juice and kept on looking for anything without high fructose corn syrup.

Boy, what a bummer! I was down to water and milk. And at that time, I hadn't gotten my fluoride water filter I talked about in the previous chapter. At that point I was starting to make it a habit to read every label. So I was wondering what poisons I was gonna find in my milk and leave me with nothing but water to drink. I tried switching to 2% milk. But it tasted weak to me. While I went back and forth between whole milk and 2% milk, I researched the information about the various types of milk. Whole milk is at least 3.25% milk fat. 2% milk is 2% milk fat. And skim and non-fat milk contain no more than 0.5% milk fat by weight. The significance of the fat content is that the growth hormones, antibiotics and other chemicals are concentrated and stored in fat cells in mammals; which includes cattle and humans. So the more fat in the milk, the more of these drugs and chemicals you will be consuming.

When you try and switch from whole milk to a lower fat milk, you will probably have a hard time and want to give up. Hey, I hope you switch overnight! But most can't do that. What I found out is that your body and mind are addicted to the chemicals you taste in whole milk. You think you like that momentary pleasure. So you have to deal with what's going on in your mind. This is true about any and every food you are addicted to. IF you crave it or make excuses for not switching to a healthier version of a product, then you are addicted to that product. I hear that about milk only second to soda pops.

Attitude and proper mind set – I want you to know that as I write this book, I have to keep trying to get the point across to you that since we all naively believe our food, drinks and water supplies are really safe...I have to work hard to get it across to you that this is absolutely false. In reality, rare few food products we ingest are safe. The FDA declares products safe as long as they don't kill you quickly. So stop agreeing to do what kills you a little bit later than if you had taken cyanide pills.

It took about 5 years of regular use of a quart of cranberry juice, 20 oz. Gatorade, 3 sodas and a quart of sweet tea a day to cause my kidney failure. And I never saw it coming. Why would I? I was eating extremely healthy and drinking Gatorade to get my electrolytes and cranberry juice full of anti-oxidants and cancer preventing Lipton sweet tea. Don't be scared. Be informed!

If I skipped all these parts about attitude and mind set, you will most likely miss the boat on actually curing yourself or preventing the diseases you will get by trusting the food companies and medical professionals. You need to have a chip on your shoulder at the grocery store that pushes you to read labels in the store and never bring the poisons home in the first place. Everything you buy is poisoned. All you CAN do is limit the amount of poisons you purchase and ingest. And when you ingest poisons in liquid form your body digests and absorbs a far greater amount of these poisons.

What about soda pops? Sorry, it's all bad news when it comes to soda pops. The acidity of all sodas is roughly 3.0. Problem is, that your body's pH needs to be between 6.0 and 7.3. The further below 7.3 you get, the more your pH adversely affects and impedes body metabolisms. In simple words, drinking sodas makes your body ripe for disease just because of the extreme acidity. The HMF in high fructose corn syrup, hydroxymethylfurfural, has been linked to DNA damage in humans. HMF content rises as high fructose corn syrup gets warm. And once it reaches 120 degrees Fahrenheit, HMF levels rise dramatically.

Then add to that the sodium benzoate that has been proven to have the ability to switch off vital parts of DNA in a cell's mitochondria. And when you add vitamin C in with the sodium benzoate it causes benzene, a known carcinogenic substance. The mitochondria is called the power station of the DNA. So this damage is severe and leads to serious cell malfunction. This damage is linked to such diseases as Parkinson's disease, many neuro-degenerative diseases and most of all the whole aging process.

Now what I am about to add about sodas is my opinion from my experiences with sodas, what I have researched and what I concluded on my own. I don't have any proof beyond my opinion and experiences. So you can choose whether to believe the following. I concluded that high fructose corn syrup mutates your genes. Some have stated that high fructose corn syrup is made with genetically altered corn in a 3 step process using genetically altered enzymes. The manufacturers of this poison won't tell you exactly how it's made and advertise what seems to be a white lie recipe for high fructose corn syrup. It shouldn't surprise anyone. They have never admitted the scientific facts about the poisons in their HFCS. They have even started calling HFCS "corn sugar" to try and hide HFCS as an ingredient in products. But it may very well be the DNA altering actions of the ingredients in sodas that I have concluded to be gene-mutating actions. I will continue being open to the facts in order to reach a final decision about this.

What is bad about sodas? DNA altering HMF, DNA altering sodium benzoate, a 3.0 acidity and possible gene-mutating high fructose corn syrup; which is also where the HMF comes from. And you get that wonderful sugar burn with every drink, and the acid also eats away at your teeth and gums. It sure didn't take any more for me to stop drinking sodas. I went from drinking at least one thousands sodas a year to somewhere around 10 to 12 sodas a year. As I look back at this, I have no doubt as to why my kidneys failed. All these serious poisons, not to mention the fact that one 12 ounce soda pop shuts down your immune system for about 6 hours. Technically it does not shut your immune system down. It's just that your immune system is pre-occupied with trying to remove all the ingredients your body can't use. That is all it can do for about six hours. Drink a soda every 6 hours and you in essence have no immune system working to heal you. How do you have a chance against sickness in this condition!

So what about tea? Tea is really good for you. I still drink tea and have all along. We switched to Lipton decaffeinated tea, but still couldn't stand swigging down all that sugar to sweeten tea. We used less and less sugar to see if that would work. You're suppose to use 4 cups per gallon. But we only used half that amount for years. So we started using less and less. It was OK in moderation, but I wasn't liking it very well after all those years of thick sugary tea. One day we heard about an herbal sweetener called Stevia. Stevia is 30 times as sweet as sugar. We used less than a teaspoon in a gallon of tea. At first I kept saying "This tea just isn't sweet at all" and started to abandon Stevia altogether. I decided that before I did that I would do a little test. So I made a gallon pitcher of tea.

I poured a few ounces into a glass, unsweetened. Then I added the Stevia to the pitcher of tea. Drank one, then the other. Ah hah! Now I could tell the Stevia really was making the tea sweet. The problem was that the tea wasn't giving my mouth that sugar burn that gives you cotton mouth, dry mouth. I then realized that I had been addicted to that sugar burn, and had been swigging down tea to get that sugar burn sensation. It's the same kind of mind addiction that all those chemicals in whole milk give you. As long as you remember that sugar burn is the proof of how bad sugar is, you will make the switch to Stevia. I'll cover this some more in the Chapter – Poisons in Your Foods, when I discuss sweeteners.

Solutions and Chapter Summary – I'm sorry to sink the Titanic about all your favorite drinks like sodas and fruit juices. But really, basically all the drink products on the market are flavored sugar waters. And most of them are packed with the worst poison of all in my experiences, research and opinion… high fructose corn syrup. You need to assume every drink product is packed with high fructose corn syrup, and check the labels to see IF you can find something that does not have HFCS.

When it comes to juices, look for products that say "NOT FROM CONCENTRATE". These words will be in plain sight. But even when the product says "NOT FROM CONCENTRATE", you still need to read the labels and see what the ingredients are. If it has high fructose corn syrup, don't buy it. The only juices we buy are Simply Orange, Florida Nature and Tropicana orange juices and Musselman's apple juice. The Tropicana orange juice in our refrigerator right now says "NEVER FROM CONCENTRATE" on the front of the cartoon. But always read the ingredients list to make sure it doesn't have HFCS in it.

That's my entire findings for juices that are worth buying, if you care anything about your health. I told you already how tiny the grocery store gets once you start reading labels to eliminate high fructose corn syrup from your diet! This is one of the main reasons I wrote this book. You can try hundreds of different juices, read hundreds of juice labels…and only about 2% of the juice products available are healthy and actually safe to drink.

In addition to Simply Orange, Florida Nature and Tropicana orange juices… and Musselman's apple juice, you can drink 2% or skim milk, Unsweetened or Stevia sweetened tea and filtered water. One juice I failed to mention was tomato juice. Tomato juice is pretty good for you. The only drawback is if you absolutely have to avoid salt, you shouldn't drink tomato juice. Tomato juice is packed heavily with salt. Tomato juice contains about 650mg of sodium per 8 ounce serving; which translates to roughly 5000mg of salt per 48 ounce can.

If you're going to drink milk, then simply drink 2% milk. If you can find it and afford it, buy Organic 2% milk. I think even Organic Whole milk would have less poisons in it than non-organic 2% milk. I drink Organic 2% milk when they have it at Kroger's. That stuff Wal-Mart sells has a slightly funky taste. That makes it suspicious to me. So I buy Organic milk only from Kroger. It's $2 a gallon more than regular milk, but well worth it. Use less milk so you buy less often. Organic milk keeps fresh weeks after regular milks have soured too.

I just recently tried that new soda pop called Sierra Mist Natural. It's a lemon lime soda that, believe it or not, does not contain high fructose corn syrup or man-made artificial sweeteners. It just contains sugar. The ingredients are carbonated water, sugar, citric acid, natural flavor and potassium citrate. Citric acid is organic. Potassium citrate is a potassium salt of citric acid. Sugar is a processed food substance and carbonated water is water that has had carbon dioxide gas under pressure dissolved in it. So that's a pretty good soda, except for the acidic carbonated water and the empty calories of the sugar. But it doesn't have a yucky chemical taste to it compared to sodas with high fructose corn syrup and sodium benzoate. That's a tremendous improvement over all other sodas. So I'll be drinking a few of them. I'll be splitting them with my wife since that's all I drink now; just half a can at a time.

Sometimes Coke and Dr. Pepper put out a limited supply of their products that substitute pure cane sugar for high fructose corn syrup. I haven't ever been able to get any. But, it's your chance to have a soda pop without that sick high fructose corn syrup or pukey aspartame or some other man-made artificial chemical sweetener.

5 -Poisons in Your Food

What do I mean by poisons in your food? I mean the chemicals that are added to food products. The most well-known are preservatives, dyes and additives of all sorts. I'm also talking about white flour, white granulated sugar, high fructose corn syrup, vegetable oils and red meat. I sometimes refer to these as poison foods. There are so many chemicals in our food supply. Quite a few of them are not necessary and are put in food products to addict you to those products. Yes, you heard me correctly.

Food companies intentionally put chemicals in your food to addict you to their products. Of course, food companies won't admit this or even talk about it. But they also never talk about any proof that their chemicals are safe. Why act like it's some secret that food companies want you to buy as much of their products as they can get you to. I've never seen any indication that they have any morals or care about you and your health one bit. All they care about is greater sales and profits to please their stockholders and their lust for money, greed. All they have to do is get FDA approval for their poisons and poison saturated products and it's all legal, approved and FDA certified safe.

As long as you don't get sick or drop dead immediately after eating their products, the FDA claims it's "safe". You are not a person or human being to corporations. You are a consumer who has what they want…your money. Has one corporation been there at the bedside of any of the millions of people their products have killed? I think NOT!

The best advice I can give anyone to inspire them to get serious about avoiding the saturation of poisons in your food is this – **Always have a chip on your shoulder when you're at the grocery store.** And no I don't mean be an a-hole to people or tackle those who look at you wrong! LOL I mean **read food labels and refuse to buy the hordes of harmful poisonous products**. I can promise you that you will begin to get furious once you start reading the labels on products after you learn about the poisons in those products.

You also need to learn what those labels mean and not be fooled by the massive trickery food companies use to trick you into buying their products. It takes more time at the grocery store, but your life is on the line and so is your health. Start right now and read all the labels on the products you already have in your home. This is exactly what my wife and I did when I blew out my kidneys in 2006.

I thought I knew the difference between healthy and harmful foods… until I started reading ALL the labels. And that was a major factor in saving my life. I'll tell you more about this later on. But for now, let's continue about food labels, what they really mean and some of the things to look for as you work to keep these poisons out of your homes and out of your bodies.

Reading labels and knowing what they mean is about the most important thing to do for finding the poisons in your food and drinks so you can avoid them.

Here's what the FDA says about the ingredient labels on products:

All the ingredients, listed in order of predominance by weight. In other words, the ingredient that weighs the most is listed first, and the ingredient that weighs the least is last.

So the first ingredient could be as much as 99% of the product. And the second ingredient could be as much as 49% of the product by weight. These are the extremes possible in any product. If a product lists any of the toxic poisons mentioned in this book in the first three ingredients, that product should be on your hit list…a product to eliminate or greatly limit and restrict its use. If the poison is toward the middle of the label, consider it a moderate health risk. If the poison is listed toward the end, consider it a mild risk if used regularly.

Reading labels MUST become a way of life. Even after years of reading labels we still make mistakes and buy products in every category; high risk, moderate and mild. IF I had it my way, food companies would be required to put labels on poison soaked products that say "Regular use of this product will cause diseases and eventually kill you." But hey, that would be honest. So that's NOT going to happen.

Take high fructose corn syrup for example: This DNA altering poison is in everything, and I mean everything. The most harmful products that contain high fructose corn syrup are fruit juices and soda pops. And yes, I said fruit juices. I don't know more harmful products than fruit juices and soda pops. They are not only saturated with poisons, as a liquid they are far more easily digested than any solid foods and therefore far more harmful. I went into some of the specific details about these drinks in the "Poisons in Your Drinks" chapter.

Now I will tackle some real problems with popular food items and tell you why you should avoid them and what you can do about substituting healthier products for those poisonous food products. Let's get started!

What about bread? Whole wheat or white? Well, the easy way is just to say eat whole wheat breads and flour. But most people don't know why they should choose whole wheat, and a lot of us can't even buy whole wheat buns, cakes, cookies, etc. You certainly can't find a restaurant that serves whole wheat bread, buns or rolls. Yes it's insane. But that's the reality we are forced to deal with. I have never understood why whole wheat bread is sometimes hard to find and nearly impossible to get in restaurants. You need to tell every restaurant you do business with that you want whole wheat bread, buns, cakes and cookies, and that you will take your business elsewhere if they don't start providing it. I doubt it will do much good, even though it's the right thing to do.

Restaurants are food companies too. So they had rather sell you white bread and vegetable oil soaked food than to take the time to care about the health and welfare of its customers. I don't believe restaurants care what customers want. At least I don't have any proof that they do. If you can find a restaurant that serves whole wheat bread or fries their foods in canola oil, then you've found a restaurant that at least cares a little about your health.

Now, what to buy at the grocery stores – If you're at the grocery store and see loaves of bread that claim they're whole wheat, look again. Look at the label. Most of what is called whole wheat is not. Food companies label it whole wheat, but when you read the label you see the first ingredient is "enriched wheat flour". Sounds good, right? WRONG!

What enriched wheat flour really is, is white flour with vitamins. What you have to look for is breads that list the first ingredient as "whole wheat flour" or "stone ground whole wheat flour". Otherwise it's only gonna be white flour in that bread. Tricky, misleading labeling is just one of the ways food corporations retain the level of poisons in food products while tricking you into believing their products are not only safe, but healthy and good for you. Nonsense!

Did you know that white flour is a drug? There is no such thing as a white flour plant. So where does white flour come from? It comes from wheat. Food companies take wheat and remove everything from the wheat that has real nutritional value and you get white flour. They remove the wheat bran and the wheat germ and end up with that drug called white flour. You can buy white flour real cheap.

Wheat bran and wheat germ are expensive and usually have to be bought from so-called health food stores; even though you can sometimes buy wheat bran and wheat germ at your grocery store. It's shocking to learn how food companies strip wheat of all its nutritional value and sell what's left, white flour. White flour eventually causes diarrhea and intestinal bleeding. This is caused by lack of fiber, and of course, if you've ever taken a slice of white bread and smashed it into as small a ball as you can, then you have already seen the proof of how white flour has no fiber. You eat the white bread and then scramble to get more fiber in your diet; when all you have to do is eat whole wheat bread and make sure it's really whole wheat. Then you would have plenty of fiber.

Trying to avoid white flour can become a real pain in the ass because of how limited the supply of real whole wheat bread is, and because of how food companies tend to rely on that drug called white flour to addict you to their products. You buy a greasy burger at a fast food restaurant and it comes on white bread so it doesn't interfere with the taste of the grease soaked burger.

Whole wheat has some nutritional value, so it also has some taste to it. You want a whole wheat cake, but can never find a whole wheat cake mix. You want whole wheat cookies, but nobody sells them. You want whole wheat buns, but you can hardly ever find them either.

So what's a person to do? You can always get a bread maker for about $70-100 and make your own. Or you can substitute whole wheat flour for white flour in recipes. You can also add some whole grains like crushed flax seed or whole wheat flour to the recipe. Adding wheat bran and wheat germ to recipes also brings some nutritional value to recipes. One thing we do is use half whole wheat flour in raisin bread. You're supposed to use bread flour. But you can use whole wheat flour as long as you add a teaspoon of wheat gluten for each cup of whole grain flour.

So when it comes to buying bread, remember to read the labels and only buy bread whose first ingredient is whole wheat flour or Stone ground whole wheat; and not to be fooled by the hordes of breads that say whole wheat on the package, but the first ingredient is white flour with vitamins; known as enriched wheat flour. There are also other whole grain breads besides wheat, like rye and multi-grain breads. When I eat out, it's at Subway's 9 times out of 10. And I always get multi-grain bread for every sandwich; not to mention the pile of chopped fresh veggies on every sandwich.

If I haven't made it clear…do not eat white bread. That means no white bread, hot dog buns, hamburger buns, dinner rolls, crescent rolls, cakes, cobblers, dough nuts, pastries and on and on and on. Look for whole wheat versions of all of these food items or do without them, or at least eat them in moderation and don't make a habit of doing so. It's not worth the damage to your health; especially when you could be eating wholesome whole grain products with the fiber and nutrients your body needs. You'll feel a lot better about yourself and enjoy a much healthier body the more you choose healthy foods, and the less you choose the unhealthy foods that the grocery store shelves are packed with. Sure you gotta spend time to learn and do all of this! But isn't your life worth the effort? Is your health worth the effort? Isn't your financial health worth it? And aren't the lives of your family and loved ones and their health and well-being worth the effort?

Making these changes in diet and lifestyle certainly is hard at first, mainly because you are so set in your ways. It's up to you to do the right thing for you and your families. I know you can do this. And the more you learn and put into practice, the more positive results you get, the more you want to learn and get to doing. And you WILL get those results as long as you make the effort.

Meat, meat and more meat – What meat should I eat? The best answer is none, you shouldn't eat meat at all. I'll go into detail about red meat in just a few minutes. But for now, let's learn something about meat in general. Meat is dead animal flesh. We fatten animals on corporate farms, feeding and injecting these animal with all kinds of drugs and chemicals, kill them systematically, skin them and cut their dead flesh into pieces and parts; which is what you buy at the grocery store.

We make up all kinds of names for these dead animal parts and flesh to try and fool ourselves into thinking we are eating something good and healthy. Millions of Americans even take dead animal parts and smoke them on their charcoal grills; saturating them with smoke and soot that tastes good, but is poison to your body. We eat the dead flesh of cows, pigs, turkeys and chickens. Quite a few people eat deer, elk, bison and an array of other dead animal flesh and parts.

Don't get me wrong. IF you can get any meat that comes from outside the corporate food companies, that meat has avoided the saturation of chemicals that are in all meat sold by corporations. You can't chase a deer down and make him drink soda pops or fruit juice to poison the deer meat. You can't inject wild deer with antibiotics and growth hormones either. The only chance of wild animals having poisons in their systems is if they have been drinking or eating chemicals that come from the massive pollution of our air, water and land by corporations.

But humans are not supposed to be meat eaters. We don't have the teeth to be meat eaters. Meat eaters have some spiked teeth so they can rip and shred meat. Humans do not. Human teeth are for chewing vegetation and fish. But no one ever talks about this, no matter how many so-called health books you read. No…we just can't bear to be honest about things. The truth might offend someone, or cut back on the sales of their book or other things. I wouldn't even begin writing this book for a few years because of that fact.

I have been attacked, slandered, hated, threatened and even had a guy pull a gun on me in Public for stating some of these facts. I have been warned by dozens of people that I am going to get someone killed by telling them how to cure themselves of diseases. All of this is insane and complete nonsense on their part. How flax seed oil, fish oil or vitamins could kill someone is unfounded and unheard of! But quite honestly, a lot of these lunatics are in the medical profession and/or their christianity has taught them to ignore God's natural cures in favor of the sorcery and quackery the medical profession invented the past 75 years. Even if there is no GOD, man has been using cures from nature since man first existed.

So telling anyone anything besides "go to the doctor" is what they pretend is me trying to get people killed. Problem with that nonsense is that I have never told anyone NOT to go to the doctor. I only tell people that IF they want to be cured, going to the doctor is not the thing to do, since doctors have no cures. If you lose your car keys, do you look on the TV and not find them and give up and never drive your car again! NO YOU DON'T. You keep looking until you find them!

And people want to accuse ME of trying to get people killed for telling you to do the same thing when it comes to your health and life! Keep going to your sorcerers disguised as doctors WHILE you cure yourself. Having a doctor to send blood tests to the lab will help you realize that you really are curing yourself, preventing disease or at the least...getting better. But I'll have a lot more to say about all this in Chapter 8. Let's get back to Poisons in our Food.

The American diet – Dead cow flesh – Everyone is on that savages' diet called the American diet; which is red meat. This country gobbles down one meal after another of that red meat that is soaked with growth hormones, antibiotics, other drugs, chemicals from the food cows eat and parasites. Red meat increases the risk of cancer, heart disease, Alzheimer's, stomach ulcers and an array of other conditions. But this country just keeps right on scarfing down the red meat. And it's the main food for almost the entire country. The fat from red meat ends up clogging your veins and arteries. This fat along with vegetable oil is the major factor in creating clogged arteries and veins and raising blood pressure by accumulating on the walls of your veins and arteries. Once this plaque breaks off it can easily lodge in your brain or heart and cause a stroke or heart attack.

I got to tell you, it just bobbles the mind how we all stuff this garbage down our own throats and no matter how many consequences we suffer for doing so, we go right on doing it day after day to no end. Why? Because we refuse to face reality as it is. So we never even think corporations would be allowed to poison everyone for any reason, including the main reason most of these poisons are in your food, drinks and water - increasing corporate profits. Your life and health are irrelevant. We are not even human beings to the corporations. We are consumers, consumers of their products. And the only thing that means to corporations is that you are the ones they work to addict to their products. And as long as you buy their products there is nothing they COULD do that would be wrong. NO WAY! Their poisons AND the products they use as the delivery device for those addicting poisons are FDA Certified safe.

All I can do is laugh at the extreme corruption of the FDA and the corporations. You need to re-evaluate your opinion of corporations who poison you in order to create changes in the human mind that cause your food addictions. As a matter of fact...all the food corporations are really doing is laughing all the way to the bank, while the medical industry laughs all the way to the bank too and thanks the food corporations for creating 75% of their business. They rake in the billions of dollars from you, while you suffer, lose your lives and end up bankrupt because of this transfer of wealth from you to the billion dollar corporations! And red meat is a major factor in all of this.

If dead cow flesh is as good for you as those who sell red meat claim, then why do you call dead cow flesh beef, steak, hamburger meat, hot dogs and all those other names substituted for dead cow flesh? It doesn't LOOK like they're trying to mislead, they ARE misleading you. Maybe if you would call something what it actually is, you might not be so quick to eat so much of it or not at all. And that's what's best for you. If you're going to eat dead cow flesh, I suggest you stick to Ground Chuck. Ground Chuck is ground beef without nearly as much fat. It's that fat, greasy taste you get addicted to eating red meat.

Now, I could go on about how bad red meat really is, but I've given you the information you need to make a rational decision to cut out red meat. If you can't cut out red meat now that you have faced the facts, then you are addicted to red meat. So to get off the red meat, you would have to pay attention to what's going on in your head while you are eating red meat. That's where the addiction is. And that's where you have to fight all these food addictions...in your head and way of thinking. Your body goes to work fighting all those chemicals and fat in red meat as soon as it gets into your body. And, your body can't rid itself of those chemicals completely under normal circumstances.

So do yourself and your own health a big favor...stop eating red meat! But since I know how hard it is to stop cold turkey, I recommend working to limit your red meat intake until you no longer eat red meat at all. I have already done this. But I do eat a pound or two of Ground Chuck in a pot of soup or a home cooked hamburger. I haven't eaten at McDonald's but once in the past 25 years, and that was when my wife and I were in Memphis for a major event. I have had my cholesterol checked and it is well within normal and I have no problems associated with cholesterol or fat. I hope you get off the red meat AND the vegetable oils that are clogging your veins and arteries and disabling and killing tens of thousands of people every year in this country.

One other tip that can help is about outdoor charcoal grilling! I use to grill outdoors every few weeks until my kidneys blew out. But that all came to a screeching halt after that happened. I love eating charcoal grilled chicken, hamburgers, steaks, hot dogs and vegetable shishkabobs. But it's easy to see why it's all bad for you. First of all, it's bad enough that you're eating dead cow flesh. But on top of the meat already being drug saturated, you smoke it with burning charcoal!

Gee, why not just stuff a wash cloth down your throat! Only difference would be the delay in taking your breath away and the time of death! Maybe you can just use the rule of doing these things in moderation and stop being so gung ho about stuffing as much red meat and charcoal grilled meat down your throat? Even the chicken, turkey and fish become repulsive to your body once they're heavily smoked on the outdoor grill.

So think about what you are really doing and stop lying to yourself about red meat being safe and smoking that meat being safe. Red meat is bad for you, and smoking it compounds that negative impact on your health. This country is obsessed with eating things that are very bad for you, while talking about the great food they are eating! This book seeks to cure you of that delusion and get you back on the road to healthy living and add days, weeks, months and years to your life and the lives of your family and other loved ones.

Vegetable oils – Canola Oil – Olive Oil or what? The simple answer to that question is olive oil. Olive oil is the best oil to use. But since it's quite costly it's not a practical solution for most people. Vegetable oils are always the cheapest. So people tend to lean heavily toward vegetable oils to cook with. But is your health and life really worth the savings in money? No it is not!

If you're old enough, you can remember how no one really said a thing about vegetable oils being bad for you until the past 20 years or less. But can you remember when no one thought cigarettes were bad for you either? Yea. **Doctors would go on TV and tell you not only that cigarettes were safe for you, but that cigarettes had quite a few health benefits.** Sounds crazy right? Totally crazy, right? It wasn't back then when they were doing this. There was no Public outcry against cigarettes at that time. People trusted their sorcerers with their new name "doctor", but not as much as people do now. They were pretty rational at that time, but were still tricked by the tobacco industry and the medical profession about cigarettes. And it's been the same story about vegetable oil and high fructose corn syrup.

You all choke down gobs and gobs of vegetable oils. It's bad enough that you cook in vegetable oil, but most of the vegetable oil you consume doesn't come from the foods soaked in vegetable oil that you fry at home. The biggest source of vegetable oils is in processed foods like Oreo cookies, Twinkies, Potato chips, breads, cakes, pies, peanut butter and margarine! I'm not picking on just these food products. The grocery store shelves are packed with vegetable oil saturated food products just like the ones I just named. You need to look for trans-fat content on the label and avoid any products that have ANY trans fats at all. In the ingredients, look for partially hydrogenated oils. Trans fats are a byproduct which is created during partial dehydrogenation.

But beware! Just because the label lists Trans fats as zero, they can still have trans fats. Food manufacturers only list trans fats above zero if the product contains at least 0.5 grams of trans fats per serving. They even fix the labeling per serving many times so they can claim their products contain zero trans fats on the label. Trans fats reduce the amount of good, HDL, cholesterol in your body. So if the ingredients list partially dehydrogenated oil of any kind, avoid that product. Do not buy it. But no matter how well you solve this problem in your own household, you still scarf down good amounts of vegetable oils when you eat any restaurant food.

There is no need to single out any one restaurant or many restaurants! Your whole problem with eating restaurant food is that none of it is healthy. They'll put out a salad bar at some places instead of cooking in canola oil, using whole wheat flour, honey and no high fructose corn syrup. They are in business to make money and make as much money as they can within the Laws of this country. The problem there is how we don't have a real government in this country any more. So it doesn't matter how bad these substances in the food supply are, as long as it's FDA approved, there is no government to do a thing about it.

Everything you eat in restaurants are cooked in vegetable oils. The damage those oils do to your body creates that craving for all the poison soaked foods and drinks you consume. It's that added taste that vegetable oils give foods that are cooked in vegetable oils. You think that chicken is good for you from that famous fried chicken restaurant, even though it's soaked in those artery clogging vegetable oils. Hey, I love their chicken. But I haven't eaten it but twice in the past four years.

About the only thing you can do about this is stop eating restaurant food; especially the big chain franchise restaurants. At smaller local restaurants you should tell the managers and owners of their restaurants that you want your food cooked in canola oil and want a better choice of drinks with no high fructose corn syrup. Let them know it's a serious health need for you and your family. But don't let anyone distract you from your choices to avoid consuming foods and drinks that are bad for your health.

The only restaurant whose food I eat is almost always SubWay. I always get my sandwiches on multi-grain bread. I usually get the Orchard Chicken. It's like a chicken salad, but has cranberries, apple and black olives on it. Of course, you can get whatever you want on your sandwich, but cranberries are only on the Orchard Chicken that I know of. I also get the Oven Roasted Chicken as my second favorite, but sometimes will get a Philly Steak and Cheese or a Meatball sandwich. Although these sandwiches aren't as healthy as the Orchard Chicken, they come topped with lots of fresh sliced veggies. And having the multi-grain bread makes SubWay the healthiest restaurant eating I know of.

I might break down once every month or two and get a Veggie Lovers pizza from Pizza Hut, but Subway is easily our favorite restaurant. I like to eat some egg rolls from the Chinese restaurants too from time to time. But hey...eating out costs at least twice as much for the same food if you cook it at home. And with the very little chance of eating anything healthy from 99% of the restaurants, eating at home is the all-around best idea for sure. So eating at home is always going to be more healthy and cheaper than any food you can get in restaurants; especially the well-known fast food chains.

Olive oil is the best oil to use by far. Extra virgin olive oil is the best olive oil. Virgin olive oil is almost as good a quality as Extra Virgin Olive oil, but is not. I always buy Extra Virgin Olive oil for about $6 a quart. My wife uses olive oil to oil the skillet to cook grilled sandwiches and other light oiling cooking jobs. You can also whip up some mayonnaise using olive oil. It will last about 2 weeks in the refrigerator. Olive oil has many health benefits which I will go in to as we go along. Olive oil even has some great health care uses I bet most of you are unaware of! Always keep some olive oil in your home, and use it efficiently to make it go a long way. If money is no object, use it generously. The more you use olive oil, the greater good you've done for yourself.

The best all-around oil is canola oil. Although it doesn't have the extensive health benefits that olive oil has, canola oil is about 25% the cost of Extra Virgin Olive Oil. Canola oil costs the same as vegetable oils. With that fact in mind, I cannot for the life of me, understand why anyone would buy vegetable oil instead of canola oil! There is no known damage which canola does to your body. On the contrary! There are lots of people who take a tablespoon or two of canola oil for their hearts most days. Canola oil has the lowest saturated fat content of all oils; including olive oil. It is very high in unsaturated fats too. Because of canola oil's excellent health benefits, I suggest you read more about canola oil and olive oil, and SEARCH the INTERNET too.

Also, peanut oil has the most (good) monounsaturated fat other than olive and canola oil. Sunflower oil is also a better choice than vegetable oils, but still lags behind olive, canola and peanut oil as far as overall health benefits. But it's still a much better choice than artery clogging vegetable oils. So avoid using vegetable oils by making the healthier choice at the grocery store. Stock up when it's on sale.

Sugars and Sweeteners – Now here's the information most people are interested in more than any other food information. It really does get confusing when you're trying to make healthy choices about sugar and other sweeteners. But just like all the food products we buy as consumers, healthy choices are hard to come by. Food companies are little to no help here either! The only healthy choices I know of among sweeteners is Stevia, raw honey and pure cane sugar. Since sugar is the most common sweetener by far, let's start there.

I told you to use pure cane sugar. But you have to pay precise attention to the term being used. You will often see, if not always, that white granulated sugar is called pure cane sugar. But it is NOT! Pure cane sugar is brown. Now you probably think you should buy brown sugar then, huh? Well don't! Brown sugar is a type of sugar. Brown sugar is just white granulated sugar sprayed with molasses. Brown sugar is NOT pure cane sugar as far as naming and labeling go. Confusing, right? Pure Cane sugar is named Pure Cane sugar and it is always BROWN. But Pure Cane sugar is not named or labeled as "brown sugar". Only buy precisely named "Pure Cane sugar" that is brown, not white.

White granulated sugar is made by processing sugar cane. They remove everything that is good in the sugar cane and end up with white granulated sugar. During that process, they add sulfur dioxide, phosphoric acid and calcium hydroxide to the liquid cane sugar that eventually becomes granulated white sugar. White sugar is toxic to your body and weakens your body's ability to fight off disease and also overloads your lymph system. Your lymph systems and nodes are part of your body's immune system. It's also a well-known fact that white granulated sugar (sucrose) causes tooth decay, and is a major factor in obesity and diabetes. I have always referred to white granulated sugar as a drug.

Many others also call it a chemical. Your body sees it as a toxin that has to be removed. White granulated sugar, sucrose, has no real nutritional value. It only gives you empty calories. And those empty calories are high octane fuel inside your body. With all that sugar firing up inside your body as instant body fuel, energy, it should come as no surprise how that process is damaging your body inside! That resulting heartburn should come as no surprise either. Hey… if you stick your hand over a fire it gets burned. Scarf down white granulated sugar and heartburn is almost certain; and more so the older you get!

Avoiding white granulated sugar, sucrose, is a pretty humongous task in this country. The only consolation to consuming white granulated sugar is that it's not high fructose corn syrup. If you just gotta eat sweets, at least make sure it does not have high fructose corn syrup! White sugar is only the lesser of two evils.

We have not bought any white granulated sugar in over four years. We do buy the brown pure can sugar from time to time. We only started doing this in the past year though. Remember, brown pure cane sugar does still have the molasses in it and is the least processed of sugar cane sugars. So it is the healthiest of the cane sugars. So if you just gotta continue with recipes that call for sugar, then substitute brown pure cane sugar for white granulated sugar in your recipes.

There are a lot of restaurants that make their own ice cream using liquid pure cane sugar. You can tell it doesn't have that sugar bite you get eating white granulated sugar and high fructose corn syrup. Brown pure cane sugar will cost you more than white granulated sugar, and it should too! Hey…you're getting sugar that has no bad health consequences, besides all those calories, and that's the most important thing when it comes to what you eat and drink.

Sometimes you can find brand named Cokes, Dr. Pepper and others that use pure cane sugar instead of high fructose corn syrup. But none of them make them a regular product you can buy year round. I've bought root beer flavored sodas, like sarsaparilla, in natural food stores, and I can tell the difference real well. But like all healthy products, they're hard to find. Healthy products will be hard to find as long as the food corporations continue to be obsessed with soaking their products with whatever poisons will addict you to their products the best.

Fructose is a better choice than white granulated sugar. Although fructose rhymes with sucrose, the name for white granulated sugar, fructose is twice as sweet per serving as sucrose. Fructose is not high fructose corn syrup either. And at this time I can't really say whether fructose is bad for you. I can only say there are healthier choices than fructose. You will find fructose in Gatorade. I keep seeing another derivative name for the sugar they put in Gatorade. So I backed off drinking Gatorade except for drinking some during hot weather.

Another familiar sweetener you see on products is Sucralose. Sucralose is the sweetener family name for a brand named product called Splenda. Although Splenda, Sucralose, is the least harmful of the man-made sweeteners, I don't use it. I don't use any of the artificial sweeteners. I have researched some other sweeteners, but haven't found any that I could trust. Aspartame is some bad crap! Some sources say that Aspartame turns to formaldehyde about 80 degrees. I don't really know, even though it's very easy for me to believe that. I'm not using any product with Aspartame in it. End of story.

Honey is another product that needs some precise information when you're buying it. You can't just pick any honey if you care about your health. You should only buy raw honey. Raw honey has not been processed. It takes honey a lot longer to start turning into a thick substance. Processed honey is always clear golden brown. Raw honey is golden brown too, but is cloudy instead of clear. Those beneficial bacteria in raw honey created this cloudiness.

Again, do your research into the many health benefits of raw honey, and do your INTERNET SEARCHes. It's hard to find raw honey in grocery stores. You should expect to pay $7 or $8 a quart when you do. I buy raw honey by the gallon for $26. It comes from a local bee farm. Use half as much raw honey as sugar if you substitute raw honey in recipes. But trying to sweeten your tea with raw honey is not really practical; although you can certainly do so if you can afford it.

When it comes to sweetening tea, we always use Stevia. Stevia is an herb that is about 30 times as sweet as sugar. Stevia has no calories too. Stevia also has no impact on diabetics, since Stevia does not affect blood sugar levels. So Stevia is an excellent healthy choice as a sweetener. When we make sweet tea at home, we use about 1/8 teaspoon per gallon of Lipton decaffeinated tea. We spend about $40 a year for enough Stevia to sweeten our tea. I drink a lot of tea, and I am thrilled to be doing so without swigging down all that white granulated sugar I drank for decades! What an improvement! If you try sweetening your tea with Stevia after having grown use to sugar sweetened tea, it won't taste very good to you at first. You won't get that sugar bite that happens to you from drinking sugar sweetened tea. So that makes you tend to think the Stevia isn't sweetening very good. What you have to do to dispel this fallacy is this:

Make your tea as you always do. Before adding the Stevia, pour 2 or 3 ounces of the unsweetened tea into a glass. Then add the Stevia to the freshly made pitcher of tea and pour some of it into a glass. Drink the unsweetened tea, then the Stevia sweetened tea. You can tell the Stevia sweetened tea IS sweetening the tea. But it's doing so without the harmful sugar bite you get from white granulated sugar, not to mention the case of "cotton mouth" you get from it! I love my Stevia sweetened tea.

I did without tea after my kidneys failed, just to avoid all that sugar in liquid form. But thanks to Stevia I've been able to drink my tea AND not have any concern about the tea doing any harm to my health. And one last thing…when I say you should drink plenty of water, that's doesn't include tea or anything that contains water. Drink all the Stevia sweetened tea you want. But don't count a bit of that tea as water.

Another sweetener you need to know about is Xylitol. Xylitol has 2/3 as many calories as white granulated sugar, but is safe for diabetics. Xylitol is found in a lot of fruits and vegetables in the fiber. Xylitol is a sugar alcohol. The most well-known use of Xylitol is for dental purposes. Xylitol kills the bacteria that cause gum disease and cavities. You will see it used in some sugarless gums too. As a matter of fact, when I get a tooth ache the first thing I do is grab a couple of Xylitol mints and slide them around the affected area and let them dissolve. It helps a great deal every time. You can get Xylitol in gum or mint form, and in toothpastes.

Eggs – There's not a lot of choices when it comes to eggs. The USDA classifies eggs as meat due to their high protein content. Just because some eggs are brown doesn't mean they are healthier than white eggs. You have to make sure those brown eggs are actually organic eggs. To comply with USDA requirements to be able to label eggs as organic, the eggs have to come from chickens that have been fed organic feed, are free of antibiotics, as well as better standards for the welfare of the chickens. The first thing you will find about the taste of organic eggs is how smooth they taste. Organic eggs don't have that chemical bite that regular eggs do. You will begin to recognize that chemical bite in regular eggs after you've eaten organic eggs for a few weeks. It's this chemical bite or burn that I focus on while I'm eating anything, in order to recognize how poisonous or healthy any food item is. I am extremely good at this.

There have been times when my wife bought some bad food product, and I used this ability and told her it has to have high fructose corn syrup. And sure enough, it does. It used to be hard for me to eat eggs. Even before I knew that bitter after taste was the chemicals in the eggs, I barely ate any eggs because of that. A better choice than regular eggs is Eggland Eggs. Eggland Eggs are organic eggs. These eggs come from chickens that are fed an organic vegetarian diet. For complete information on Eggland Eggs visit

http://www.egglandsbest.com/egglands-eggs/faq/our-eggs.aspx

In this book so far I have touched on the tricks food corporations use to trick you into buying their products. Some of the most popular labeling scams are using terms such as Low fat, Low salt, Low Calorie, Organic, All Natural, Diet and From Concentrate. But as you'll find out, these terms are misleading and downright false as common sense goes. Take the Low fat, Low calorie and Low salt labeling scam. If a product contains all three of these ingredients and advertises one of these terms on the label, then the label is correct and legal. So no problem, right?

No, you are wrong! If a product label says Low Salt, but has sugar and fat in it too, the food companies add about twice as much sugar and fat as the regular version of the same product! But hey, at least they didn't lie on the label. They just didn't tell you on the label that it also had twice as much sugar and fat too! LOL You should read the label of the regular version of any product and compare it to the Low fat, Low calorie and/or Low Salt version of that product to confirm these facts. When I first started trying to avoid salt and sugar, I read hundreds of labels of products using these labeling terms and 100% of them confirmed these facts for me. I then ceased to buy any and all products with these labeling terms and so did some friends of mine.

So unless you have some specific condition that requires you to avoid salt, sugar or fat, then stick to buying the regular versions of these products. But make sure the regular version is a healthy choice…or never put it in your grocery basket and bring it home. That's where the front line on healthy eating and avoiding poisons is…right there in the grocery store reading those labels.

Don't be fooled by other labeling tricks either, like Organic. I've pointed out some places you can trust the organic label term. But often times, organic doesn't mean organic. And it's left up to each one of us to sort this trickery out for ourselves. The same is true about the labeling terms Natural and All

Natural. You also see the term natural ingredients as well, to convey a meaning of healthy food. But with all these terms, even the ingredients listed on the label itself will give you the proof to contradict these terms on most of these food and drink products.

You begin to find out what the food companies are pretending to be natural in their tiny world. Rare few of us would ever agree with the vast majority of the food and drinks corporations' idea of natural, All Natural and natural ingredients! **And these misleading labeling terms are fooling lots of you into continuing to use the same unhealthy products you always buy, by including one of these new misleading label marketing tricks/terms.**

But in spite of all of this, you still have that wonderful fruit juice you love to drink. Yea, it's the one that says "Contains 100% Fruit Juice". I'm laughing now as I do just about every time I see that term on a product. If it's "100% Fruit Juice", then it contains ONLY fruit juice, right? Nope. Again…Read the label and see if the juice is the only ingredient. If not, you have your proof about this misleading labeling term. When I see that term I always think "Yea, I bet you took a little bit of "100% Fruit Juice" and put it in that product. But what's all that other crap in there!"

Don't forget the whole wheat labeling trick where they call their products whole wheat by using white flour enriched with vitamins. Only buy those that say whole wheat flour or stoned ground whole wheat flour. Buy the brown pure cane sugar, not the white granulated sugar labeled as pure cane sugar. Don't be fooled by the new term for high fructose corn syrup, which is "corn sugar". They just changed the name…even though I had such wonderful (sarcastically saying) things to say about corn sugar under its real name – high fructose corn syrup…like this.…

It's just an adorable name…high…oh yes, I love to be high… fructose…ahh, it's SO SO SWEET…corn…yummy yummy corn… syrup…so thick and sweet, like me! Ba hum bug. Gag me with that poison and blow out my kidneys and almost kill me. Not so uplifting, sweet, yummy thick a product as the name implies. It should be called HFCS, Heinous Freakin' Causer of Sickness!

There has been lots of information about the negative effects of MSG, but food companies continue to use MSG. So you have to read the labels and do not buy products with MSG. Food manufacturers try to hide the fact that their products contain MSG by listing ingredients that contain MSG, but not the MSG itself. So avoid products if they contain free glutamate to insure your best possibility of avoiding MSG. Besides MSG, there are thousands of chemicals in food and drink products. My aim was to focus on how to reduce the total amount of poisons entering your body.

This is why I am not including a long drawn out explanation about the many other poisons in your food and drinks, or in our water supplies and personal hygiene items. I have given you a powerful guide that will result in you reducing the amount of poisons getting into your body. Remember, it's toxins, also known as free radicals and poisons, that cause almost all disease. So eliminating poisons is reduces the amount of disease your body develops.

I've even heard doctors state the fact that toxins, free radicals, cause many diseases. I just haven't ever seen a doctor with the desire to trace that toxin back to its source. As sad as it actually is, your doctor can't make no money if he solves that problem; cures that disease by eliminating the poisons causing the disease or condition.

It's all up to each of you to use the power of knowledge in order to find your way through all the deceit that hurts us, but can't do a thing to change these food and drinks corporations. And that's what this book can do for you...guide you through all the things that stand in your way, to keep you eating according to corporate advertising and misleading labeling, and the most important facts you need to make the serious changes concerning all the products you buy that you consume. I will not suggest that you try to talk with any of the food corporations or anyone in the government in pursuit of solving or diminishing this plague of poison induced sickness and disease affecting every human and animal in this country. Our humanity limits us time wise.

So use your time to read labels while you are in the grocery store. Work on recognizing the foods your mind craves when you are addicted to a food product. You have to understand that you can't wipe out all the poisons overnight! You have to start somewhere and keep learning progressively. Search the INTERNET for lots and lots of information on every subject and item. Look for information that repeats itself time after time while you're doing your searches and research. Cut back on eating out to avoid eating unhealthy. Cut down on charcoal grilling and the amount of meat you grill each time. The less poisons you put in to your body, the less health problems you will have.

I also didn't spend time going over the details of the benefits of eating fresh fruits and vegetables. To me, that's real simple. Eat all the fresh fruits and vegetables you can. Just make sure you wash them real good. I even take each grape I eat and wipe it off real good with a paper towel.

To see for yourself what good this does, eat a few grapes and focus on the taste. Then wipe off a few grapes with a paper towel and eat them. Then eat some grapes without wiping them off and notice that slight bitter taste each grape has. That's the poisons the grapes are soaked in that you are tasting.

Wash fruit and vegetables extra good and eat all you want. Buy organic produce to reduce those poisons as much as possible. And, Buy fresh over frozen, and frozen over canned.

6 - What Else You Can Do To Speed Your Healing

I know that was a lot to take in about all the poisons in your water, drinks and food products, and the excessive obsession corporations have with deceiving you and addicting you to the chemicals they saturate all their products with. That is why I often told you to use Chapters 3, 4 and 5 as guide from now on. Judge your water, drinks and food according to what is stated in those chapters. This book is about YOU being cured. YOU getting better. I'm not against doctors. I am FOR people and living things being well and free of disease.

I don't allow my thoughts to be filtered through money, religion, politics, opinions or anything else. I had to become that way to save my own life. Everything I shared in this book is to help you and help you return to making cures a part of Life; instead of remaining in that hopeless abyss under the helm of doctors.

When it comes to doctors and this country's medical profession, they are the best doctors in the world in emergencies. But when it comes to disease, they are among the worst doctors in the world. And when you are dying, you don't have time to be distracted with what a bunch of cold hearted greedy bastards doctors are. You have got to focus on doing everything you can to get better and save your own life. And even if this cure for cancer was not true, most of us believe that we don't just lay down and die. We try to Live as long as we can, and will fight as hard as we need to, in order to extend the time of our precious lives.

When I started doing these things myself, I didn't have a single thought of me curing myself of arthritis. Or a single thought about curing myself of heart disease. Or curing myself of headaches, heartburn, bleeding gums, intestinal bleeding or even dandruff! All I was trying to do was extend my life a little beyond the 2-3 years doctors gave me before I would be dead or on dialysis. So I know you gotta be a bit skeptical that our food, drinks and water supplies are making us all sick and killing us years before our time. But it's true. And no corporation is going to remove those addicting poisons they saturate our food, drinks and water with.

So it's all up to YOU to learn how to avoid their poisons. YOUR life depends on it. So you DO have the time to learn these things and save your own life. Then spread this knowledge to others until it spreads like wildfire; on the way back to normal thinking and way of living.

There are other things that are known to help people with cancer. But before I get to that, here's some information about one of the most common forms of cancer, breast cancer.

Breast Cancer - It's a scientific fact that flax seed oil kills breast cancer cells at least as fast as chemical therapy, but without all the pain, suffering, hair loss and huge medical bills as the medical profession's artificial chemotherapy. If you had been on a proper human diet of fish, you most likely wouldn't have gotten breast cancer in the first place. The omega-3 fat, alpha-linolenic acid, found in flax seed and walnuts and cold water fish like tuna and salmon, provide the best protection against breast cancer. Studies have shown that women with higher omega-3 content in their breasts had the lowest risk of breast cancer. It's pretty much common knowledge that a woman's breast is mostly fatty tissue.

And with all the omega-6 rich vegetable oils you consume combined with the low levels of omega-3 in the normal red meat American savage diet, that throws the healthy ratio of omega-6 to omega-3 fats way out of ratio. This creates a disease ripe environment for breast cancer and other cancers. Add to that, all the poisons you have yet to recognize and avoid, is it any wonder why you have breast cancer!

Since many breast cancers depend on estrogen, you should take Calcium D-Glucarate; which helps the body excrete used hormones such as estrogen. Calcium D-Glucarate is known to remove, detoxify, cancer causing carcinogens in the colon, skin, liver, breasts and lungs. Do not confuse Calcium D-Glucarate with any other form of calcium. Buy only products that state the term Calcium D-Glucarate clearly and specifically. Calcium D-Glucarate is found in many fruits and vegetables, but one 500mg tablet of Calcium D-Glucarate contains as much phytonutrient as 82 pounds of fresh fruit and vegetables.

And don't forget the anti-oxidants either; Vitamin C, A and Selenium to remove toxins and Vitamin E to help speed along your healing of damaged cells. Cancer is caused by damage to the nucleus of cells. This damage interferes with apoptosis, which is the natural programmed death of cells. When this process breaks down, cancer cells begin to form. Cancer cells do not experience programmed death as normal cells do. This allows cancer cells to grow and divide; which leads to a mass of abnormal cells that grows out of control and forms tumors. Once these tumors form, they develop blood vessels. These blood vessels carry cancer cells to other parts of the body and form growths.

The damage to cells is caused by gene mutations causing cells to be unable to correct DNA damage. Cancer is a result of these mutations which interfere with oncogene and tumor suppression gene function and leads to this uncontrollable cell growth. Carcinogens are directly responsible for damaging DNA and promoting cancer. Free radicals are formed when our bodies are exposed to carcinogens. These free radicals damage cells and inhibit normal cell function. If your family members have had cancer, especially your parents and grandparents, it's obvious this gene mutation was passed on to you. But even so, this only means cancer forms quicker in these people than those without the family history of cancer. And as soon as your body is exposed to carcinogens, cancer begins to form.

You should also avoid smoking and excess exposure to the sun. Since free radicals cause cell damage, you should take all the anti-oxidants you can. Take the prevention/maintenance dose if you don't already have cancer. If you already have cancer, take mega doses of vitamin C. A mega dose would be at least 5000mg daily, and as much as 10,000mg daily. Also double the maintenance dose of Vitamin E, A and selenium and take around 100mg of Alpha Lipoic Acid most days to boost the effectiveness of those anti-oxidants. Take fish oil or flax seed oil too, as recommended earlier in this book; since both are anti-inflammatory and help create balance with omega-6, to prevent and cure disease.

Your immune system controls cancer cells in your body. You rarely have a problem with cancer as long as your immune system is healthy. Your immune system works to remove toxins to keep you healthy. Take Astragalus and even dandelion root to boost your immune system. Take 1000-3000mg daily for 2-3 weeks, then 1000mg Astragalus every other day or few days

As you may recall, I also pointed out earlier in this book that sodium benzoate and high fructose corn syrup cause DNA damage. So anything with either of these should be high on your list of poisons to eliminate. Soda pops have both of these poisons. And much to my surprise, Mrs. Weavers sandwich spreads have sodium benzoate. So we rarely ever buy Mrs. Weaver's pimento, chicken or ham sandwich spreads. I always loved her products too. This is why you read the labels before buying any product. It takes valuable time out of our busy lives, but is THE KEY in avoiding products with these poisons.

Don't make the mistake I did, and do this AFTER you are already sick. Which would you choose........? Having cancer and wishing you had've taken the time to read the labels and avoided getting cancer or some other disease? OR Taking the time to read the labels and avoid the cancer altogether? **Living this chronic delusion that poisons are safe as long as they're in our food, drinks, hygiene items and water supplies.....is the problem this book cures. Once this problem is solved so that poisons are bad for you; ESPECIALLY when those poisons are in your food, drinks and water, disease will fade to the background** and most of us can die like most people use to........of old age; not disease. And cancer will cease taking our loved ones prematurely!

I am always amazed at how even though toxins, aka poisons and free radicals, cause cancer, I haven't heard about any doctor telling anyone to get rid of the poisons that caused their cancer. That is, beyond saying to stop smoking! But you can keep right on obeying your doctor and paying those high medical bills WHILE you cure yourself naturally and without all that suffering and pain.

Some other things that can help cancer patients are Astragalus, Cayenne, Garlic; as well as Vitamin C, Calcium, Fish Oil, Flax seed Oil, Lemon Balm, Sage, Vitamin D and Calcium D-Glucarate. Let's take a closer look at these Vitamins, Herbs and Food substances.

Astragalus - Astragalus is an adaptoge, meaning it helps protect the body against various stresses; including physical, mental, or emotional stress. Astragalus may help protect the body from diseases such as cancer and diabetes. It contains antioxidants, which protect cells against damage caused by free radicals, byproducts of cellular energy. Astragalus is used to protect and support the immune system, for preventing colds and upper respiratory infections, to lower blood pressure, to treat diabetes, and to protect the liver.

Astragalus has antibacterial and anti-inflammatory properties. It is sometimes used topically for wounds. In addition, studies have shown that Astragalus has antiviral properties and stimulates the immune system, suggesting that it is indeed effective at preventing colds.

In the United States, researchers have investigated Astragalus as a possible treatment for people whose immune systems have been compromised by chemotherapy or radiation. In these studies, Astragalus supplements have been shown to speed recovery and extend life expectancy. Research on using Astragalus for people with AIDS has produced inconclusive results.

Recent research in China indicates that Astragalus may offer antioxidant benefits to people with severe forms of heart disease, relieving symptoms and improving heart function. At low-to-moderate doses, Astragalus has few side effects, although it does interact with a number of other herbs and prescription medications. Astragalus may also have mild diuretic (rids the body of excess fluid) activity.

Traditional uses include the treatment of the following: Stress - Colds and influenza - Persistent infection – Fever - Multiple allergies - Asthma - Chronic fatigue - Fatigue or lack of appetite associated with chemotherapy - Anemia – Wounds - Heart disease - Kidney disease – Hepatitis - Stomach ulcers - Diarrhea – Stomach Gas – Bloating

Vitamin C – An antioxidant, Vitamin C prevents the free-radical damage that contributes to aging and aging-related diseases, including cancer, cardiovascular disorders and others.

A major contributor to our immune system, Vitamin C helps increase resistance to a range of diseases, including cancer. Excess Vitamin C stimulates the production of lymphocytes, an important component of our immune system. Ascorbic Acid is also required by the thymus gland, one of the major glands involved in immunity, and increases the mobility of the phagocytes, the type of cell that "eats" bacteria, viral cells, and cancer cells, as well as other harmful invaders.

Vitamin C acts in many ways to help prevent high blood pressure and atherosclerosis; hardening of the arteries that can lead to heart attack and stroke.

Vitamin C forms cementing substances, such as collagen that hold body cells together, thus strengthening blood vessels. Hastens healing of wounds and bones and increases resistance to infection. Aids in the utilization of iron. Converts Folic Acid into its active form. Increases our ability to absorb and store iron. Improves the bio-availability of selenium.

Vitamin C is used by the liver to detoxify drugs and other chemicals, and appears to protect the body from the side effects that accompany many drugs. Another important role of Vitamin C is the one it plays in our ability to handle all types of physical & mental stress.

To prevent colds, in August start taking 1000mg of Vitamin C as cold and flu season approaches. Keep this up all through the cold and flu season to prevent colds and flus. If you already have a cold or get one any way, then take 1000mg Vitamin C every 4-6 hours until you are well; usually 3-4 days later instead of 10-14 or more. Vitamin C is an essential nutrient and is also called ascorbic acid, L-ascorbic acid and L-ascorbate, and should not be confused with citric acid. You will sometimes see it used in food items. Since your body doesn't store Vitamin C, it's up to you to make sure you take Vitamin C supplements. Vitamin C is inexpensive too. Vitamin C was the first vitamin to be mass produced back in 1934, when it was artificially produced and marketed as Redoxon.

Here is a table for suggested Vitamin C dosage for specific conditions:

Condition	Suggested dosage in mg
allergies or asthma	3,000-7,000
bleeding gums	1,000-3,000
cancer prevention	5,000-10,000
coronary heart disease prevention	500-4,000
enhanced immunity	1,000-5,000
exposure to cigarette smoke & polluted air	1,000-5,000
high levels of stress	1,000-5,000
surgery, wounds, injuries	5,000-10,000

Calcium – Calcium is found in every cell in your body. So its importance is obvious. Calcium is used to build strong bones and teeth, where almost all the body's calcium is stored. You need a minimum of 1000mg of calcium daily. It is very important to note that calcium will cause you problems like bladder and kidney stones, and bone spurs, if you don't take magnesium supplements. It takes magnesium to dissolve the calcium to make calcium of use to your body. Without enough magnesium to do this, calcium particles are able to bind with toxins to form bladder stones, kidney stones and bone spurs. Calcium causes your heart to contract, while magnesium causes your heart to relax; thus creating proper heart rhythm.

Calcium has been found to lower blood pressure, lower risk of colon and prostate cancer and prevents osteoporosis. You have four parathyroid glands on the back of your thyroid gland that regulate the amount of calcium in the blood and bones. Besides taking magnesium with calcium, you should also be sure to take Vitamin D; especially during winter when you don't get much sun.

Calcium D-Glucarate – Calcium D-Glucarate is the calcium salt of D-glucaric acid, and is found naturally in the body. Since many breast cancers depend on estrogen, you should take Calcium D-Glucarate; which helps the body excrete used hormones such as estrogen. Calcium D-Glucarate is known to remove, detoxify, cancer causing carcinogens in the colon, skin, liver, breasts and lungs. Do not confuse Calcium D-Glucarate with any other form of calcium. Buy only products that state the term Calcium D-Glucarate clearly and specifically. Calcium D-Glucarate is found in many fruits and vegetables, but one 500mg tablet of Calcium D-Glucarate contains as much phytonutrient as 82 pounds of fresh fruit and vegetable.

Men may want to take Calcium D-Glucarate to help remove excess estrogen as part of your cure for erectile dysfunction. Women should take Calcium D-Glucartate to help relieve symptoms of menopause and menstrual cycles, because of its effectiveness in removing used hormones such as estrogen.

Cayenne – Cayenne, or cayenne pepper, is one of the most beneficial foods around. Cayenne pepper can bring amazing results for simple healing and challenging health problems. It has been scientifically proven that Cayenne pepper kills prostate cancer cells. It can stop heart attacks, help rebuild flesh harmed or destroyed by frost bite, heal stomach ulcers, rebuild stomach tissue and heal hemorrhoids. In your circulatory system, cayenne improves blood circulation, rebuilds blood cells, lowers cholesterol, emulsifies triglycerides, removes toxins from the blood stream and overall improves the health of your heart; as well your blood pressure.

Cayenne can also heal your gall bladder and remove plaque from your artery walls. It has also been known to be an effective diuretic and help in both urine elimination and built up fecal matter in the intestines. There is so much to say about cayenne peppers. The reason you don't hear about this powerful healing medicine is that the medical profession is in the business of making money, not healing people. If they were, cayenne pepper would be at the top of their list. But, they haven't even mentioned it yet!

Vitamin D – Vitamin D is a powerful cancer preventative. Vitamin D activates your immune system to fight rogue cancer cells; as well as normalizing and correcting cancer cells. Vitamin D also plays an important role in preventing any kind of disease. The best way to get enough Vitamin D is to spend an hour in the sunshine each day. Take Vitamin D supplements the days you don't. Vitamin D can change most everything in cancer cells; including its genetic messaging and its cytoskeleton (cellular structure); which is made out of protein. Vitamin D keeps cancer from spreading by reducing cell division, and can return a cancer cell to a normal healthy state. All of these facts are major steps in beating cancer. So make sure Vitamin D is one of the top items on your list of things to take daily.

Fish oil - Fish oil and omega-3 are known to have many health benefits. As a matter of fact, I have mentioned fish oil many times in this book, because the so-called American diet is so deficient in omega-3 that almost every person in this country suffers the effects of not being on a fish diet as man is suppose to be. Fish oils contain the omega-3 fatty acids eicosapentaenoic acid (EPA), and docosahexaenoic acid (DHA), precursors of eicosanoids that are known to reduce inflammation throughout the body. Fish oil comes from the tissues of oily fish such as cod, haddock, salmon, trout, sardine, herring and mackerel. Fish oil is high in Vitamins A and D and omega-3 fatty acids. Its most well-known benefits are in helping those with heart disease, depression and inflammatory conditions such as arthritis. Fish oil is an anti-inflammatory.

Some of the conditions that fish oil cures, prevents or improves are depression, peptic ulcers, Alzheimer's disease, Chron's disease, Colitis, Breast Cancer, lupus and heart disease. Fish oil also improves your skin, promotes weight loss, prevents schizophrenia, eases bi-polar disorders, improves brain function, increases eye focus and much more. The EFAs, essential fatty acids, in fish oil fight the plaque in the brain that causes Alzheimer's. Those already afflicted with Alzheimer's disease can reduce the symptoms of Alzheimer's.

Fish oil emulsifies the plaque that clings to your artery and blood vessel walls, which causes high blood pressure, hardening of the arteries, heart attacks and strokes. It acts like a scavenger to clean your blood and make your blood flow more smoothly. It also cures arthritis by lubricating the joints and acting as an anti-inflammatory to reduce the pain and swelling associated with arthritis. Fish oil is also beneficial to the pancreas and strengthens a weak pancreas and is a strong ally against cancer of the pancreas.

Fish oil is proven to prevent breast cancer, as well as cure breast cancer. It kills breast cancer cells as fast as chemotherapy. This is because of the high fat content in women's breasts; which almost every woman is seriously deficient in, due to not being on a fish diet.

Out of all the deficiencies in your diet, the lack of omega-3 is the most problematic of all deficiencies; followed by magnesium. That is why I suggested every one take fish oil and magnesium as their first items to take; after you get that water filter for your kitchen and shower. I take fish oil, flax seed oil and other oils containing EFAs like Primrose oil and Extra Virgin Olive oil. Primrose oil contains GLA; which is the most biologically active form of Omega-6 fatty acid.

You can get good quality fish oil at Puritan's Pride. The particular fish oil we buy is found at **http://www.puritan.com/nutritional-oils-068/omega-3-fish-oil-1200-mg-013326?NewPage=1** .

If you have any chronic disease or condition, take 3000-5000mg fish oil daily for 3-6 weeks, then back off to a maintenance dose of 1000-1200mg daily or most days. If this does not cure a disease or condition known to be cured by fish oil, then take the larger dose several weeks longer.

And make sure you do your own research to find out all the different diseases and medical conditions that fish oil helps. There's so much more to learn than what I have included in this book. But merely taking fish oil as an all-around preventative is one of the very smartest things you can do for your health.

Flax seed – Flax seed is the vegetable form of omega-3; whereas fish oil is the animal form. Flax seed oil can be used in place of fish oil, but the combination of the two seem to provide the greatest benefits. So the same things said about fish oil above, are also true about flax seed and flax seed oil; though flax seed oil is the most beneficial in preventing and curing breast cancer.

Garlic – Garlic is one of the most potent natural medicines of all time. It contains over 400 health enhancing chemical compounds; making it an all-natural medicinal treasure chest. The most powerful compound from garlic is allicin. Allicin is produced when garlic is chopped or crushed. So the more crushing or chopping, the more allicin is generated; thus increasing the medicinal effect. Allicin has an excellent antibiotic, anti-fungal ability. Powerful sulfur compounds in garlic kill and inhibit an amazing array of fungi, viruses, molds, bacteria; and even worms and parasites. Among the things garlic can do is lower cholesterol and blood sugar, detoxifies, strengthens the immune system, inhibits cancer, treats HIV/AIDS infections, fights respiratory diseases, lowers blood pressure and kills herpes on contact.

Garlic has been known for its healing powers for several thousand years. It's best to eat garlic raw, crushed or chopped. But a lot of people prefer to take garlic oil capsules. Dry garlic tablets are the least desirable. Take 1000mg daily as a preventative, and 3000-5000mg for 3-6 weeks if you have a disease or condition which garlic is known to cure or help. I haven't ever heard of anyone having adverse effects from garlic, except for having occasional "garlic breath".

Garlic needs to stay high on your list of healing foods; along with fish oil. The Garlic we buy is at Puritan's Pride at **http://www.puritan.com/garlic-060/garlic-oil-1000-mg-002970?NewPage=1#product**

Lemon Balm – Lemon Balm is a perennial herb in the mint family. Lemon balm, along with chamomile, were used as "cure alls" by ancient Egyptians. The health benefits of lemon balm include improvement of digestion and memory. Lemon balm leaves are abundant in certain chemicals, such as protocatechuic, rosmarinic and caffeic acid, flavonoids and phenolic compounds, which in turn contribute to the various health benefits. Research has confirmed the antioxidant activity of lemon balm extract. It also decreases the risk of cancer. Lemon Balm, Melissa officinalis, plays a vital role in the treatment of hyperactivity, a common disorder in children.

Distraction, hyperactivity and impulsiveness are the three common features of the Attention Deficit Hyperactivity Disorder (ADHD). A significant improvement in the memory performance and cognitive functioning is seen to be associated with supplementation with dried lemon balm leaf. Certain individuals with dyspepsia are seen to improve with a supplement of lemon balm, in combination with peppermint, licorice root, caraway and candytuft.

Leaves of lemon balm can play an important role in the treatment of flu, lowering of blood pressure, improving memory, releasing of certain hormones, treatment of depression and thyroid and relief of insomnia or sleeplessness. Lemon balm tea is useful for thyroid problems. Grave's disease is a condition associated with the excessive production of the thyroid hormone. It is an autoimmune disorder and lemon balm decreases the secretion of the thyroid hormone. Lemon balm is also used as a nerve tonic. It also relaxes the muscles of the bladder, stomach and uterus.

This may explain what I was feeling when I drank lemon balm tea the week my kidneys blew out and I was pissing blood and blood clots. The lemon balm tea went down my throat and immediately began giving me a warm relaxed feeling in my throat, which spread and flowed to my stomach and intestines. I stopped pissing blood after drinking lemon balm tea. I figured it was proving itself as the "cure all" Egyptians believed it is.

Lemon balm is also good at relieving headaches, and is effective against herpes simplex, dementia, Alzheimer's disease, lip sores and spasms. Its antiseptic properties make it good for treating allergies, acne and skin rashes.

Lemon balm is also good for keeping insects and flies away and out of your house. Just clean your kitchen and toilet seats with an infusion of lemon balm to keep the bugs away. And of course, you can use lemon balm to add lemon flavor to any dish like fish or Bar-B-Q meat and chicken. Lemon balm goes well with allspice, mint, pepper, rosemary and thyme.

Sage – Sage has the broadest range of medicinal uses of all herbs. Sage is anti-inflammatory, anti-microbial, anti-hypertensive anti-diabetic and cleanses your blood. Sage is also known to prevent Alzheimer's disease. Sage was used as a cure all by Native American Indians and still is. No matter what ailed them, drinking sage tea was a major player in recovery from those ailments. Sage is another great asset in your efforts to overcome cancer; just like Vitamin D. And as with everything, I urge you to do Internet Searches for Sage and all these herbs, vitamins and food substances. Stick to the positive information though; since doctors who claim to know nothing about herbs, vitamins and food substances have begun to claim they are experts on how no vitamins, herbs or food substances can help you in getting over any disease.

Sage can also ease and cure bleeding ulcers and repair your stomach and intestinal walls. But in general, Sage is an antispasmodic, antiseptic, astringent, bitter tonic and stimulant. Sage is used as a throat and mouth wash you use by making a strong tea and gargling with it. For ages, sage has been used in treatments for disorders involving the gastrointestinal tract. Sage helps to relieve muscle spasms in the digestive region and it is also been used as a cure for indigestion. It has also been known to help lower blood sugar levels in diabetics. It is also a fact that sage helps to improve memory and brain function. When used in combination with rosemary and ginkgo biloba, it is thought to help prevent and even slow down the progression of Alzheimer's.

And as a precaution, remember to avoid large doses of Sage if you have high blood pressure, epilepsy or kidney disease. The same is true about licorice. And **always put a good meal or at least one hour between doses of herbs and vitamins, and any doses of drugs you take. The Vitamins and Herbs are completely safe. But those drugs doctors prescribe kill over 25,000 Americans every year.**

Sage is known for its flavor on turkey and turkey stuffing. Sage has also been used for sore throats, eye infections, gum disease, weak appetite, menopausal hot flashes and excessive sweating, infertility, tonsillitis and mouth sores and ulcers. Sage is also used externally for wounds.

Sage is originally from the Mediterranean region but is widely grown in sunny locations with well-drained soil. Grow your own herbs and include Sage, so that you will have fresh live Sage to use to provide the health benefits it is known to provide you. Cut the Sage and dry it at the end the growing season. Cut the plant back to about one third its size and hang the branches upside down and bundled together. Once it dries naturally in a few days, strip the leaves off the branches and store it in vacuum sealed jars, bags or canisters. Make sure to add some Sage to your soups and stews too.

And you should take as many additional anti-oxidants as you are willing to take. I don't mean huge doses. I mean, willing to take daily for a few months. Then continue taking them several times weekly the rest of your life. Some of the anti-oxidants besides Vitamin C, are Vitamin E, Vitamin A, Selenium and Alpha Lipoic Acid. All remove the toxins that cause cancer. And Selenium is a very potent anti-cancer agent.

There are also large amounts of other anti-oxidants in Goji berries, Mangosteen and Noni. It is these extremely powerful anti-oxidants in high amounts that bring the claims of miracle healings by drinking the pure juices of Goji berries, as well as Mangosteen and Noni fruit. I highly recommend the pure forms of these. But you should never believe any ONE thing is going to cure you. It's the total amount of poisons that enter your body, not any ONE poison, or any ONE diet deficiency.

Now, here's a short summary of what you should focus on eating.

The Best Things to Eat to Help Cure Cancer

Now that you have read what you have to know in order to cure yourself, or at least significantly improve your health, I'll give you a short summary of what foods you should eat. This book focuses on reading labels to recognize the saturation of poisons in our food, drinks and water supplies, NOT a special diet you can follow to cure yourself. Technically, there isn't a special diet you can go on to cure any disease. Your diseases are caused by poisons. Anything that your body naturally removes is considered to be a toxin. That includes all man-made chemicals that enter your body through your mouth, nose, eyes, lungs, veins, pores or otherwise.

But there ARE foods that are more beneficial to people with cancer, than other foods are. Earlier in this book I told you what I consider to be The Perfect Diet. But The Perfect Diet is The Perfect Diet for people in general, and best for the overall best health of people. But if you want to focus on the most beneficial foods for speeding your healing, here's what you should focus on:

Eat oily fish like salmon, herring and mackerel and others. Cat fish is not one of them. Cod and Tilapia are other good choices.

Stick to colorful fruits and vegetables such as carrots, peppers, pumpkins, cabbage, broccoli, Brussels sprouts, eggplant, tomatoes, apricots, cherries and red grapes. If the fruit or vegetable is purple, you can count on it being a strong agent against cancer.

Eat Mushrooms, Garlic, lentils, chick peas, soya, Brazil nuts, Pumpkin seeds and Sunflower seeds. All of these inhibit cancer cell growth,

protects the immune system from toxins and stops the spread of cancer.

As important as this information is, I chose to simplify it as much as I can. The big job is trying to find something to eat in the grocery store that is NOT packed with disease causing poisons. And when you do that, the grocery store becomes a very tiny tiny place. You are tempted to continue buying the crap that made you sick and is taking your life away from you. It takes some hard work and time to make the transition from debauchery to caring about your own health and life.

Debauchery is defined as extreme indulgence in sensual pleasures. And that is exactly why you are sick. Food corporations work to addict you to their products by adding substances like high fructose corn syrup in excessive amounts to addict your brain with an addiction that affects the brain the exact same way cocaine does. You sit in the kitchen smacking on that sugary snack, cake, cookies and pies; washing it down with soda pops or fruit juices. You're 30-100 pounds overweight. You know you shouldn't be eating that crap! So WHY ARE YOU?

That's how you behave when you are addicted. It's the behavior of people who are addicted to the saturation of poisons in whole milk; the growth hormones, anti-biotics and all the other drugs cows are routinely injected with. Not to mention the poisons in that dead grain most cows are fed. You have got to face the fact that you are addicted to these poisons, so you can do something about it.

None of the food and drink corporations are going to remove their poisons. You have to deal with reality as it is; not how it SHOULD be. **If you're gonna depend on the corporations to remove the poisons that made you sick, then you have no hope whatsoever.** This book is about empowering YOU with the knowledge to cure yourself of cancer and all disease, by doing something to avoid the poisons that cause all disease. I don't want you to forget that your attitude and state of mind have to change before your health can change. I cannot cure you. And no doctor can cure you either.

YOU are the one who can cure YOU. And this book was written to provide you the information you must know in order to cure yourself, or at least significantly improve your health. You cannot eat those poisonous foods I just mentioned and expect to cure your cancer. It wasn't lack of fresh fruits and vegetables that made you sick. It was poisons, toxins, chemicals that made you sick. And the only way you are going to cure or prevent disease is by avoiding the poisons that cause all disease.

So this is the end of the information you need to cure yourself. But make sure you go ahead and read the next Chapter for My Final Words. I saved some interesting facts for the end of the book. And of course, there are other things that help cancer patients. But I have covered the knowledge and proven science that will cure you or at least improve your health significantly. I have said this more than once in this book. Why didn't I say everyone will be completely cured?

I don't know all the 100's of millions of circumstances in people's lives. So there is no way I can determine the outcome in ALL those people's lives. **What I can do and did do in this book is give you the written knowledge of proven science which doctors intentionally ignore in order to prolong your illness to maximize their income.** But I did not waste my time trying to change doctors or the helpless medical profession! It's for that same reason I've said before; that poisons caused your disease, not lack of fruits and vegetables. And it wasn't for lack of doctors or nurses. And it wasn't caused by lack of exercise. Your cancer and all disease is caused by POISONS. And since it's those poisons that cause all disease, it's those poisons you gotta concentrate on avoiding, in order for your health to recover and make you well again.

And now that I have given you all the information you need to guide you in healing yourself as fast as you want to, I have a few things to tell you that I believe you need to be aware of, about your cancer, all diseases, doctors and the medical profession, food and drink corporations and a few things about me and how I discovered the scientific cure for cancer. It's the information up to this point in the book that will save your life. But let me tell you a few things before we end this book, in the final chapter, My Final Words.

The Cure For Cancer

7 - My Final Words

Here we are at the end of the book. I know you have learned a lot of things you did not know. The trick is to put the information to use so that your cure can be a reality and not just hope. I just can't stress it enough about poisons causing your diseases! So buying all the cancer diet books can help, but they are not the cure for cancer. The cure for cancer is to get rid of the CAUSE of all cancer. And the cause of all cancer is poisons.

It's like your floor being flooded with water. If you're a doctor, you charge us to mop up the water again and again. But a plumber finds the CAUSE of the leak and fixes the CAUSE of the leak in order to stop the consequences of the leak. So I cannot take credit for this common sense fact that we all know as humans. Find the cause. Get rid of the cause and you get rid of the problem, the disease. But how is it that I know the cure for cancer?

After doctors told me I would be dead or on dialysis by 2008 and would not do anything to help me get better, much less cure me, I started looking for anything that MIGHT help my kidneys get better. I had arthritis, bleeding gums, intestinal bleeding, headaches, heartburn and a few other diseases for at least 20 years. I had headaches from time to time my whole life. So I sure never gave one second of thought to curing myself of any of those conditions. All I was trying to do was help my kidneys and hope I could add some time on to the short time I had left to live. And even after curing myself of chronic bladder stones in 1996, what I was about to do would end up shocking even me! It all began when my 84 year old mother was in Intensive Care in St Bernard's hospital.

I was talking to the head nurse in the Intensive Care wing at St. Bernard's, when she told me her husband also had kidney disease. I asked her what he was doing about it. She told me he was using ginger packs placed on his kidney area. These ginger packs soak poisons out of the kidneys. And since no one had told me anything that could help me, I was anxious to get some ginger root and start using these ginger packs.

But as I was looking for the ginger roots, I began thinking that you wouldn't have to soak the poisons OUT of your kidneys, if you didn't put those poisons IN your kidneys in the first place. Then, I wondered why anyone would put poisons IN their bodies in the first place. I also wondered what and where the poisons were coming from that caused my chronic kidney disease. And the intense search and activities began!

I began to examine everything I ate, drank or came into contact with. The first thing I did was buy a fluoride water filter to replace our Water Pik faucet end filter. Then I bought a shower filter. I also quit using the microwave to cook, and began using it only to heat things up no more than 30 seconds. I couldn't find much wrong with what I was eating; except for some red meat. But when I began to examine what I was DRINKING, boy did the scum rise to the top in plain view!

And once I found that damned high fructose corn syrup saturating my fruit juices and soda pops, I began finding it in almost everything. I did some tests to see what was causing me to get all tense. And I kept getting that tense feeling every time I consumed something with high fructose corn syrup in it. And the more a product had, the more tense it made me.

So I began avoiding the products with high fructose corn syrup in them. There goes my Kraft Bar-BQ sauces, mayonnaise, ketchup, ice cream, bread and on and on and on. Boy, when you begin to look, you soon learn that once you get rid of the products saturated with high fructose corn syrup, there's barely anything left in the grocery store you CAN buy. And now, the heartless bastards that make this poison are running commercials claiming your body sees high fructose the same as sugar. My response is "My body never did. Your high fructose corn syrup almost killed me." And I am not looking for revenge against these killers.

I am looking to save people from these killers and their saturation of addicting drugs they saturate all their products with. Their response is to claim their products are safe like the FDA says. And that normal use of their products will NOT make you sick or kill you. But then you have THEM as the proof that they work hard and spend billions of dollars in advertising to entice you to consume large amounts of their poison saturated products! And the rare times "government" does their job to govern these poison peddlers, you have all these whackos claiming their Rights are being violated by the government NOT allowing them to buy excessive amounts of these corporations' poisons!

Now ordinarily, I would agree when government prevents you from doing something you choose. But, when the City of New York banned sugary drinks over 16 ounces, they were not violating anyone's Rights. They were and are, forcing these poison peddling corporations to stop pushing their poison saturated drinks on the people in excessive amounts. The wrongs of these corporations are being limited, or governed, for the safety and well-being of The People. And this IS the real role of government. The most important part of this is that, gene mutated high fructose corn syrup should already be banned. If it's just like any other sugar, then why is high fructose corn syrup the only sugar made from genetically altered corn and genetically altered enzymes?!?

Once I began to eliminate the high fructose corn syrup, things started changing for the better with me. It was the first thing I knew was actually helping. And in this book, I have told you all the things I did to help myself and cure myself of chronic kidney disease and at least 7 other chronic diseases and medical conditions. That was every disease and medical condition I had. When all I was trying to do was help my kidneys get better to add a little time to my life, past the 2008-2009 time doctors said I would be dead or on dialysis. I was so amazed at what happened, it took a while to sink in. I figured since there were no cures for any of these chronic incurable diseases I had, that I was probably just fooling myself while my diseases were actually getting worse.

But after a few years I began to accept the fact that I was actually cured of all those things. No more headaches, heartburn, arthritis, kidney problems, intestinal bleeding, bleeding gums or anything else. So as the days, weeks, months and a few years passed, it slowly began to sink in that I am actually cured of all this. It's weird never having a headache. I haven't had a headache since early 2007, after having 2 or 3 a week for the past 20+ years; same as with the heartburn, bleeding gums, intestinal bleeding and arthritis.

I decided to write a book to share as much knowledge as I could, in order to help as many people as possible. The book focused on chronic kidney disease, but is titled "Self-Care HealthCare Guide". I worked hard on that book and tried to keep it as a guide for curing yourself of everything I cured myself of. I realized that once I finished that book, it contained the cures for most diseases specifically. But even though the book was finished, I continued doing some research about other major diseases like cancer and liver disease and a few others. What I found out is that, one after another after another disease is caused by poisons. Fact is, 80% of all disease is caused by poisons. The other 20% is caused by germs or viruses. All cancers are caused by poisons. But diseases such as hepatitis are caused by a virus. So I took those facts and back tracked them.

My book is about avoiding the poisons that cause all these chronic diseases. All cancers are caused by poisons. So there is your cure for cancer. I was really in shock for a few weeks and thought about all this over and over and over. And the more I thought about it, the more it excited me. I wasn't looking for the cure for cancer, much less the cure for all chronic disease. But I lived it, THEN realized what I had actually done. It took me over a year to start thinking about writing this book, since I had already given the cures for every chronic disease in my first book, Self-Care HealthCare Guide. I even added "BOOK of CURES" to the title. But no one bought the book after that either. That's why I took the cure for all disease from Self-Care HealthCare Guide and directed the attention on one disease, instead of all disease, for this book and another book I wrote titled How to Avoid Dialysis and Cure Kidney Disease.

It is real frustrating to have such great and powerful knowledge and have it almost completely ignored. But no one is picking on just me! The one doctor who I found is keeping people off dialysis, is being ignored too; Dr. David Moskowitz. He is talked about in depth in Self-Care HealthCare Guide and also in How to Avoid Dialysis and Cure Kidney Disease.

Dr. Moskowitz turned over his proven treatments to arrest kidney disease, to the National Institute of Health. It is their job to get this information to this nation's medical profession to put into practice. But even though Dr. Moskowitz's treatment would have saved the government $500 Billion in just the past 10 years alone, to this day, the NIH claims they don't even know about Dr. Moskowitz's treatments and don't even know what they are.

And before that, the VA hospital Dr. Moskowitz worked at and had kept over 1000 US War Veterans off dialysis for up to 11 years, put an end to Dr. Moskowitz's treatments. And one by one they all got worse and worse, to the point that Dr. Moskowitz could not bear to continue watching it. So he resigned from that VA hospital. And when my doctors began to realize that I was curing myself, they sent me certified letters stating that they would no longer be my doctors. They were quite nasty about it when I called them to ask what was really going on with all that.

Never depend on the doctors or medical profession to cure you. Doctors never studied cures and never studied medicine either. As a matter of fact, doctors abandoned all cures and medicine in the entire history of man, starting about 75-100 years ago. Use doctors and the medical profession for what they DO.

They're real good at doing tests and diagnosing disease, prescription drugs, surgeries, medical procedures and for emergencies. But when it comes to curing disease, the doctors in this country are among the worst in the world. This is why this nation's sick care "health care" system is only the 34th best care in the world, while being #1 in cost of that care.

So whether you listen to doctors or not, one thing is certain. The only way you have a chance of being cured is IF you cure yourself. Or maybe you think I have a chip on my shoulder just because this cure for cancer and most all disease is being ignored by the medical profession? My response to that would be "I'm not a 17 year old girl or a researcher at the University of Canada at Alberta either." So you might think "Terry, are you crazy? What does a 17 year old girl and researchers in Canada have to do with this cure for cancer being ignored?"

Uh, I'm the one telling you the cure for cancer. But no one listens. But no one is listening to the 17 year old girl. The one I'm talking about is Angela Zhang, who attends Monta Vista High School in California. She started developing a cure for cancer when she was 15. Angela had an idea to mix cancer medicine in a polymer that would attach to nanoparticles that would then attach to cancer cells, which would show up on an MRI. She then aimed infrared light at the tumors to melt the polymer and release the cancer medicine. This proved to kill cancer cells while leaving healthy cells unharmed. And what about "researchers in Canada"?

Researchers at the University of Alberta in Canada discovered a simple, inexpensive drug that is proven to kill cancer cells. The drug is called dichloroacetate (DCA). DCA changes the metabolism of cancer cells and causes them to age and die, a feat that is alien to cancer cells and stops them from otherwise destroying the human body. This drug has been around for quite some time, and was proven to kill cancer cells in 2007.

But it has been held up with a lot of testing, and is not being funded very well. This is going on with a drug that can very well bring an end to cancer. So regardless of who has a cure for cancer or any disease, all cures are being ignored by the medical profession; even when a cure comes from one of their own.

But there's one thing I want to tell you about before I end this book. It's about how radical I have been all these years in my knowledge of natural cures and medicines.

It wasn't too long ago that I happened to catch a CBS episode of 60 Minutes. I saw them advertise that program and didn't want to watch it because I knew they would just say how stupid all of us are for saying anything bad about sugar, and especially that sick crap known as high fructose corn syrup. But my wife and I sat and watched the show, knowing what they were gonna do. The only hope was that Dr. Sanjay Gupta was hosting the segment we wanted to watch. I kept the remote in my hand, ready to turn it, to keep from hearing their nonsense. But as it turns out, I got a big surprise from that segment.

Dr. Robert Lustig of the University of California at San Francisco is called a pioneer in what some call the war against sugar. The main diseases Dr. Lustig says are linked to sugar are type II Diabetes, Obesity, Hypertension and Heart disease. He says the American lifestyle is killing us and at least 75% of it is preventable. Dr. Lustig has published at least a dozen articles on the evils of sugar. But the way most people heard what he had to say was through his video on You Tube called Sugar: The Bitter Truth. Dr. Lustig and I are in agreement on everything except one point.

He says high fructose corn syrup is no worse than any other sugar. He does admit that it's the fructose that we crave, because there is fructose in every fruit; but not in the high amounts as in high fructose corn syrup. And in fruits, that fructose is diluted by water, fiber and nutrients. That's why consuming fructose in fruits is the way to have a balanced diet. But when we consume high fructose corn syrup, it doesn't seem bad at all, since we were born to love fructose, in all our fruits, naturally.

In that same report, they told about a nutritional biologist at the University of California Davis, who conducted a 5 year study linking excessive high fructose corn syrup consumption to diseases such as heart disease and stroke. Her study showed that calories from high fructose corn syrup effected the body differently than calories from other sources. She used a completely controlled environment in her study.

Her subjects were in a kind of 24 hour lock down. Everything they ate was weighed and calories counted. They began eating normal meals, then began adding sugar in their diets so that 25% of their calories were from sugar. And in just two weeks, the ones who got 25% of their calories from high fructose corn syrup, had higher levels of bad cholesterol, LDL and other increased indicators of cardiovascular disease.

What they discovered was that when your liver gets overloaded with fructose, it begins converting it to fat, which produces LDL; which forms the plaque that clogs your arteries and blood vessels.

Their report also included some information on research studying the effects of sugar, glucose, on cancer cells. Cancer cells feed and grow by hijacking the flow of glucose in your blood stream. This is especially true with cancers known to have insulin receptors. And then there was the guy who did CAT scans on the brains of humans to see the effects of high fructose corn syrup on the brain.

He found out that high fructose corn syrup affects the brain in the same way as cocaine does. Dr. Sanjay Gupta volunteered to have the CAT scans done while he was given a sip of soda pop through a tube. The CAT scan showed blood flow increased to certain parts of the brain as the soda hit his tongue. His brain began to release dopamine, as though it was some kind of addictive drug. The person conducting these tests on hundreds of people is Eric Stice, a Neuro Scientist at the Oregon Research Institute. He concluded that as you eat more and more sugar, your body builds a tolerance to it. That causes you to crave more and more sugar as this tolerance level increases over time. This is exactly what happens when you are addicted to drugs. And that brings me to the strangest part of that segment. Actually it was the only strange part to me.

At one point, Dr. Sanjay Gupta is talking to this Dr. Lustig, the guy they said was leading the war on sugar, and Sanjay asks Dr. Lustig if he is going to go out on a limb and say that sugar is a toxin, a poison. Well, Dr. Lustig said he believes it is. But what about ME? I didn't go out on a limb recently and say sugar is a poison. No, that was Dr. Lustig.

I'm the guy who not only went out on a limb and said sugar is a poison. I said white granulated sugar is a drug. I didn't go out on a limb saying that. I rode a rocket ship off THAT limb. And I rode a rocket ship off that

limb back at least 30 years ago; about 1981. So I was really thrilled to see this doctor and these scientists presenting solid scientific evidence to back up what I began saying 30 years ago. And in that segment, they also let one of those guilt ridden sugar cane farmers TRY to defend his crap.

Now, let's get this straight from the beginning. This sugar cane farmer could have just said that he grows the sugar cane. And it's not his fault that corporations take his natural sugar cane and make the drug called white granulated sugar, instead of making pure cane sugar. But he actually tried to defend this crap. And this is the pathetic destructive mentality that develops when all anyone cares about is money. His sugar cane is good. Taking it and making drugs from it is what is wrong, wrong, wrong, wrong, wrong! But even though I appreciated that fine segment from CBS 60 Minutes, I had an alarmingly negative experience with one of their employees, former Miss America Debbye Turner.

Debbye grew up in the same city I did. Her grandmother lived across the street from us, and remained our neighbor when we moved a block away from her. So Debbye and I were "Friends" on FB. I had spoken to her in person before. But she is younger than me. So I didn't know her very well. One day Debbye makes a post on Facebook about a CBS news story she was doing, about looking for a cure for cancer. So I commented on her post and gave her the cure for cancer. It was actually an abbreviated explanation, and I also mentioned the cure was in my book Self-Care HealthCare Guide. I also offered it for free to all my Facebook friends. But after a couple of hours, no one had said anything in response to my comments. I couldn't find my comments. So I made another post asking why Debbye deleted my comments. And her reply even shocked me. And I can tell you plenty of things I have witnessed that would shock almost everyone. And only a tiny bit of that really shocks me.

Debbye said she was not going to tolerate hate speech from anybody. And before I could ask her what she was talking about, Debbye went ahead and said she was talking about me posting the cure for cancer on her post! As ridiculous as that was, I could only believe she was joking at that moment. But she kept on with that, and even got a couple of people to support her on her bold statement that posting the cure for cancer is "hate speech". But that time with Debbye Turner was not the only time the haters have lashed out at me for saying there is a cure for cancer. But why did I share this with you? What good does it do to tell me all of this, you might ask.

I want you to cure yourself while you listen to your doctors, so you don't get all scared a lot of the time while you wait for your cure to become obvious. I wish I could tell you that your doctors, family and friends will support you in your efforts to cure yourself. But it's just not what I am able to tell you. Everyone will tell you to only listen to your doctors. And it won't matter that the doctors sentenced you to death. It won't matter that without a cure you are dead!

Thinking outside that tiny bubble about your health that doctors created over the past 75-100 years, is not something you are going to find support for. Even when you are advised to talk to your doctor before taking any herbal medications, they know that only a rare few doctors will say anything true or positive about anything that they don't make money off of. If doctors could patent Vitamin C, they would have gladly told you that Vitamin C cures the common cold. But since no one has a patent on Vitamin C, we're told there IS no cure for the common cold.

But no matter how hard doctors and the medical profession and drug companies ignore natural substances in favor of their artificial substitutes for most all natural substances, you still need a cure for your cancer. And that is THE most important thing. So DO what I laid out in this book. And use Chapters 3, 4 and 5 as a daily guide to eliminate or at least greatly reduce the amount of poisons going into your body. Your health will change for the better. Those changes for the better will become noticeable within a few weeks. And as those changes in your health for the better continue to increase over the next months, your goal of curing yourself of cancer will become a reality to you.

The cure for cancer is not really a secret. I have seen plenty of cases of people curing themselves of cancer on the VERIA TV network. There were several people with stage 4 cancer who cured themselves doing an important part of what I tell you to do in this book; which is making the effort to change to what I call The Perfect Diet. One woman I remember, had just a few months to live and was also pregnant. And she is still telling her story here 30 years later. She gave birth to a son too. She turned a horrible horrible situation into the most wonderful event in her life, by believing she COULD be cured, and dwelling on natural things instead of the artificial means provided by this nation's medical profession.

So let me remind you one more time about WHAT a cure is. A cure is the thing that saves you from sickness and gives you Life instead of Death. In my world, cures are second only to family and living things in importance. If I had rode the pony the doctors gave me to ride, I would be dead, and there would be no books from me to help anyone. So cures are HUGE in my world. I have come to realize that even though cures have been ignored by the general Public over the past 75 years that more and more people just want to be cured.

And since doctors have no cures, you are only going to find out about these cures from someone like me. You can also check historical facts, like reading up on Hippocrates, the Father of Medicine. Then you will know doctors do

NOTHING Hippocrates did. But it's all good news to everyone BUT the medical profession.

About half of what I told you in this book closely resembles holistic medicine. That's because the cure for cancer and all disease, deals with your whole body problem. Your cancer doesn't come by itself. No disease comes by itself. So treating symptoms is only good for prolonging your disease and running up all those medical bills that bankrupt a million Americans each year. But the most important facts for being cured are not taught in holistic medicine. And that is the part about the poisons that cause all disease, except for the 20% caused by germs and viruses. I saturated my kidneys with poisons that no one BUT me had ever called poisons. And I did so to the point that my kidneys turned to mush and failed, with my blood pressure going sky high to 240/140 for several months. All due to the fact that your liver converts excess high fructose corn syrup to fats that become LDL in your blood stream.

There are cures for every disease. But they're all outside the medical profession. And when it comes to cancer, no doctor is gonna turn his back on all that money those chemotherapy drugs make them in favor of telling you that poisons caused your cancer, so you can do something about that problem. But that's actually perfect with me. Why? Because I am a pure American. So I know the U.S. Constitution does two main things. One is to establish Individual Rights as the Supreme Authority of America. And even in the bible, Christ Jesus died so that each Individual could receive all that GOD has for you (His Holy Spirit) without any connection to any group or christian church.

And when it comes to any possibility of you being cured, yes sir, yes mam! It's YOU, the Individual, that can save your own life, the lives of your loved ones; cure yourselves, and make cures a part of your Life again. I cannot cure you and no doctor can cure you. YOU can cure YOU! That is so wonderful and Powerful, and even more so when you compare that to the hopelessness of the helpless medical profession. But continue looking for any signs of progress toward cures.

If you search for a cure, you will find it. And you have found the cure you were looking for right here. You can cure yourself WHILE you still listen to your doctors, except about death and there being no cure. And you can do it for very little money. And best of all, it all depends on YOU. This book contains the knowledge to empower YOU to cure yourself. You must DO what this book says. And the more you do what this book says to do, the faster you will get positive results, and those results will be more and more significant as you do more and more of what this book teaches you to do.

The point you want to get to is when you have learned to buy groceries and have read the labels on every product so many times, that you only bring home a tiny bit of poisonous crap or have made the decision to leave the crap alone altogether. And you have gotten use to drinking your pure clean water as an essential habit to maintain good health. You are going to have to make a lifestyle change. And I don't mean you have to give up your life. I mean that, now you know that all the food in restaurants are bad for you, are you going to stop eating out as much as you have and only do so rarely.

Or you just gonna keep on like you have been, down the path that led to you getting cancer. I get kinda of skiddish when friends suggest I come over and eat with them. It's like my high school class reunions. There's no way I would eat the crap food you eat! All smoked meats and all of it red meat except for some chicken wings is what I see as stupidity in relevance to eating healthy.

So you are going to have to make those lifestyle changes to sustain your cure and good health once it is restored. But while you work on that, make sure you focus on avoiding the poisons that saturate our entire food, drinks and water supplies. Because those poisons are the cause of your diseases. I would wish you luck with doing what my book says. But it's all science. You don't need luck with science. You just use the science as it is. And that's what this book is about; the proven science about what causes all disease and how to recognize those poisons so you can avoid them, and all the chronic diseases that they cause.

And last of all......If you think you can really trust your doctor, who is supposed to BE a Physician by definition, yet cures no one, just remember that back a few decades ago, doctors were on TV not only assuring the Public that cigarettes are not bad for them, but that smoking cigarettes had various health "benefits". Then maybe you can get on over that hump of believing in death sayeth the doctors, and getting on with curing yourself because that's what you want. That's what your family wants for you. And a cure is the only thing that is going to save your life.

I wish all of you the very best in your efforts and congratulate you on what you are about to discover; something that doctors say does not exist - the cure for cancer and the world where that cure and all cures come from. It's the world you lived in as a child, but turned your back on once you got all grown up and didn't have to listen to anybody and nobody could tell you what to do any more. And now it's time to be a child again, and allow the power of knowledge to heal you and set you free of that world of hopelessness cancer and all disease bring.

And may this saving knowledge reach all your loved ones and reach around the world to open the eyes of all who seek a cure for their cancer and other chronic diseases. Cures are here to stay. Embrace them and hold on to them as an important part of Life. Be safe. Be well. Love and Peace to everyone.

DISCLAIMER

This book was written to guide people in doing the things that will improve their health and cure them if they are willing to do the natural things it takes to do so. While there are some facts stated in here that are critical of some things, there is absolutely no intent to defame or misrepresent the facts about these persons, companies or others. On the contrary, I intentionally left out the names of the companies saturating our food, drinks and water supplies. I did this so that no one would think that talking to these people or companies is of any real value.

So, if anyone takes anything said in this book to mean to defame, misrepresent or anything of that nature, they are only stating their opinion of what is in the book, but not stating an opinion based on facts.

I am fully aware of how the people in the medical profession, generally and according to my own experiences, will attack and criticize anything that is not something they do and make money off of. I have no interest in their drama and choose to avoid it altogether. I have never told anyone to stop going to the doctor. On the contrary, I tell them to cure themselves WHILE they still do what the doctors say to do. I'm not afraid of doctors. I just know not to look to doctors or the medical profession for cures.

No one should, in any way, take anything stated in this book as promoting or even suggesting any type of action toward any part of government, companies or the likes. On the contrary, I suggest you stop buying products with the disease causing poisons pointed out in this book. And no one should be so twisted and perverted in their minds to claim that we as Individuals do not have the Right to protect ourselves from disease causing poisons, and all poisons.

This book places absolutely ZERO HOPE that food, drinks and water companies will ever make the choices to remove the poisons from their products. So, the only choice we have is to freely share the knowledge individuals need to avoid the poisons in food and drink products, as well as the water. Just because doctors and the rest of the medical profession don't get to make money off the diseases I cure or prevent and never have, doesn't constitute any illegal or inappropriate act or acts.

There are only a rare few places in this book where any text was copied or paraphrased from a web site for this book. These few places were from Public sites with no copyright stated. This was only done for accuracy of facts, rules and policies. Anyone who thinks their copyright has been violated in any way, can contact me for a quick and amicable solution in your favor.

There is nothing in this book that could be construed as being illegal, libelous or defamatory. I didn't go into the facts about how food and drink corporations deliberately formulate addicting drugs and poisons to saturate their products with. I assumed you have the sense to know all these food and drink corporations know they are doing this, doing it deliberately and using the FDA as their save all entity, to save them from their own fraud, deceit and intentional harm to the health of most people who consume their poisons.

In other words, no matter how harmful the poisons these habitual criminals put in your food, drinks and water are, they always spout how all their products are FDA approved and certified safe. And it is YOUR place to tell yourself that these poisons are NOT safe, no matter what corrupt propaganda the FDA spouts.

I will state unequivocally, that those in the FDA belong in prison to await their execution for their Treason against The People of the United States of America. They have betrayed the Trust of The People habitually, and their habitual Treason has to be stopped. And even though the food and drink corporations can hide behind the FDA, The People can put a stop to this poisoning The People to Death; just to maximize the profits of the corporations the FDA protects with their massive and habitual deceit.

It is my basic Constitutional Right to criticize the government. And without the habitual, massive fraud of the FDA, the rate of Death by chronic disease, and the huge number of people with chronic diseases, would decrease and fade back to being a noticeable problem instead of the overwhelmingly plague that it is. And the systematic plague the food and drink corporations perpetuate with the help of the FDA, would finally come to an end. And this blood thirsty sick care medical profession in this country would be DE-throned. And people would slowly return to acting sane and normal, and take care of their own health, with cures returning to being THE essential and most important service doctors provide.

In the bible, it says "Physician, Heal thy self." It says that because healing is the place of a Physician. I wonder IF any of us will see any doctor turn their backs on this modern medicine sorcery as their only methods, and get back to being Physicians, healers, in our life time. It's a far-fetched notion. But until doctors begin to make that choice one day, the only Physicians the world is going to have is people like you and me.

Be Well. Be Cured, but don't be fooled by doctors with no cures!

Alphabetical Index